MAGNETIC RESONANCE ANGIOGRAPHY BASICS TO FUTURE

Edited by **Wael Shabana**

Magnetic Resonance Angiography Basics to Future
Edited by Wael Shabana

Published by InTech
Janeza Trdine 9, 51000 Rijeka, Croatia

Publishing Process Manager Bojan Rafaj

Technical Editor Teodora Smiljanic

Cover Designer InTech Design Team

Additional hard copies can be obtained from orders@intechopen.com

Magnetic Resonance Angiography Basics to Future, Edited by Wael Shabana
p. cm.
ISBN 978-953-51-0401-8

For EU product safety concerns:
IN TECH d.o.o., Prolaz Marije Krucifikse Kozulić 3, 51000 Rijeka, Croatia,
info@intechopen.com or visit our website at intechopen.com.

Meet the editor

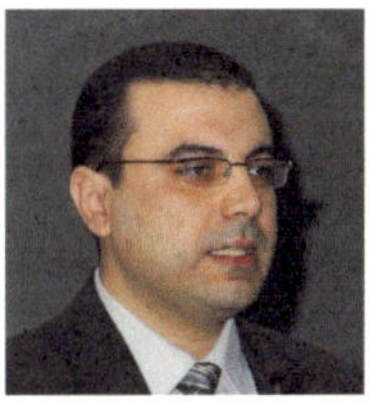

Wael Shabana finished the first medical school (MBBCH) in Egypt. He gained Master in Medical sciences from the Free University of Brussels, (VUB) Belgium. He had the second medical school in Belgium from the VUB with distinguishing degree (MD). He did his residency in the university hospitals of VUB (UZ- VUB). He gained successfully PhD during his residency from the VUB. He did a fellowship in abdominal imaging and cross imaging intervention in University of Michigan -Ann Arbor. He joined as a staff in U. Mich- Ann Arbor , before he joined University of Ottawa as assistant professor. He has interest in applied clinical research, MRI research and other fields in radiology.

Contents

Preface

Diagnostic radiology had significantly changed the practice in the medical field in general, and in surgery in particular surgery. It shaped the pre-treatment and pre intervention planning which improved patient selection, treatment selection and outcome. Radiology also allowed a more objective evaluation of treatment and treatment effects. The same role is played by MRI in the field of angiography. MRI angiography hand in hand with CT angiography established an important role as a diagnostic modality that is equivalent to the conventional diagnostic angiography. This geared the interventional angiography towards more therapeutic role. Leaving the diagnosis, pretreatment mapping to MRA as a subsequent to the road map defined by the MRA. The pre-treatment road mapping had significantly impacted the patient outcome. Which is the ultimate goal. MRA has the potential of providing more physiological and pathophysiological data over the disease in addition to the anatomical information.

This book is divided into three sections. The first section discusses the basics of MRI angiography. The first chapter focus mainly on the contrast agents that are mainly used in MR angiography with detailed discussion of advantage and limitations of different types of contrast. The second chapter is oriented more towards the technical consideration that contribute to good quality examination, both the non contrast and contrast based sequences from black to bright blood imaging, contrast agents, review of clinical application of MRA in different body systems and MR venography.

Section two is covering the advances in the head and neck, brain ischemia imaging. A review of the advances in intracranial plaque imaging with High-resolution magnetic resonance imaging can identify plaques on the arterial wall as well the plaque instability. The future prospective of such technique as well the limitation are discussed. Further points of discussion like pathophysiological advantage of MR in understanding the mechanism of hemodynamic of brain ischemia, the intracranial atherosclerotic stock as well the future challenges and clinical implication of MR in this field. The quantitative MRA analysis is a new technology that provides non invasive method to measure the blood flow in the brain. An over view and presentation of technique is covered in the last chapter of this section

In section three, emphasize the use of MRA in the aortic and peripheral vascular disease in pediatric population.

I would like to thank my colleagues who contributed to this work and who invested their time in bringing that work to light. We as a team hope that this book will be provide added knowledge to the field of radiology. I would like to thank the publisher who allows the transfer of this knowledge and make it available as an open source to everyone who is interested in the field. Hope you will enjoy reading this book.

Dr. Wael Shabana, MD, PhD, Assistant Professor,
Department of Diagnostic imaging, University of Ottawa,
Canada

Part 1

Basics and Applications of MR Angiography

1

MR Angiography

Brian Ghoshhajra, Leif-Christopher Engel and T. Gregory Walker
Harvard Medical School / Massachusetts General Hospital
Boston, MA,
USA

1. Introduction

Diagnostic angiography was first performed in humans by Moniz in 1927 (Nath 2006), but did not achieve widespread adoption until Seldinger facilitated a safer method via flexible catheter access rather than direct needle access in 1953(Seldinger 1953). Since that time, invasive diagnostic angiography enjoyed rapid adoption, with further therapeutic interventions now performed in nearly every vascular bed. In 1974, the first reports of magnetic resonance imaging (MRI) were published(Macovski 2009), which soon added to the arsenal of the radiologist's tools to image the body and eventually its vessels. In recent years, noninvasive imaging (via ultrasound, x-ray computed tomography [CT], and MRI) has decreased the frequency of diagnostic angiography which is in many cases now reserved for high-risk patients, and situations with a certain or high likelihood of intervention (Saloner 1995). While the role of the diagnostic radiologist has therefore been redefined, this development has also contributed to the rise of subspecialisation in the field of interventional radiology, via improved planning and post-procedure management. Today magnetic resonance angiography (MRA) is widely available, and is the standard of care for many diagnoses in the neurologic system, and is rapidly becoming a first-line test in many centers for peripheral vascular imaging, imaging of the great vessels, and in some cases can even be applied to the beating heart, allowing noninvasive coronary MR angiography for selected applications. This chapter will review the basic forms of MRA as organized by pulse sequences and image types (technical considerations), and then review examples of these techniques as performed in each body system.

2. Technical considerations in MR Angiography

From its inception, MRI has allowed imaging of the vessels, by virtue of its cross-sectional nature. Although MRI initially presented an advantage over CT by its unlimited imaging planes, the advent of multidetector CT with isotropic resolution has slightly dampened this enthusiasm. MRI does however, enjoy the advantage of its lack of ionizing radiation, relative freedom to image large patients without image compromise, and ability to repeat acquisitions when necessary. Ultrasound remains the first line test for imaging flow velocity, but MRI can indeed quantitate blood flows and velocity with technically advanced sequences.

This section will first review the non-contrast enhanced (non-enhanced) techniques for imaging vessels, followed by pulse sequences requiring intravenous contrast. Image post-processing techniques for vascular imaging will briefly be reviewed. Contrast agents themselves, and relevant safety issues, will then be reviewed.

2.1 Non-enhanced MRA

Non-enhanced MRA can be achieved because the magnetic properties of flowing blood are inherently different than that of stationary tissue. This ranges from relatively simple "black blood" techniques, to phase-contrast imaging, and relatively modern inflow techniques. These techniques are advantageous because they do not require intravenous access, and can be repeated if necessary. They may be less robust for imaging diminutive vessels, and depending on the pulse sequence, may not be available on all scanners.

2.1.1 Black-blood techniques

Black blood techniques are produced via pulse sequences that null the signal from moving blood. While they are relatively simple (based upon spin echo techniques), they can take relatively long times to acquire. More recently fast spin-echo and single-shot techniques have decreased acquisition times. Although they are widely available and relatively robust, these techniques are often supplanted by more advanced pulse sequences. However, in cardiac imaging, they remain a basic staple, particularly when coupled with nulling techniques that decrease the signal from moving blood. Black blood techniques also are advantageous when imaging of surrounding soft tissue anatomy is desired. (Lee 2005)

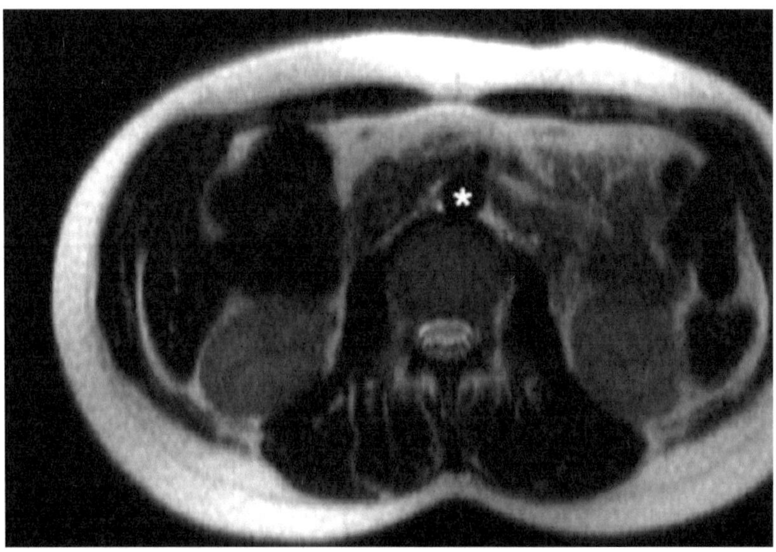

Fig. 1. Black blood effect. Fast spin-echo T2-weighted axial MRI image demonstrates a normal flow void within the abdominal aorta (asterisk). This pulse sequence can be obtained on any modern scanner, and takes advantage of the inherent lack of contrast in a flowing vascular bed when performing basic spin-echo acquisitions.

2.1.2 Bright-blood techniques

Gradient-recalled echo techniques improve dramatically the speed of acquisition that MRA can be performed. More modern iterations include balanced steady-state free precession imaging (aka. "white blood"), and have allowed cardiac MRI with cine imaging to be robust enough for routine use. These sequences can be used for localization and imaging of surrounding tissues (although they are less reliable for tissue characterization). (Lee 2005)

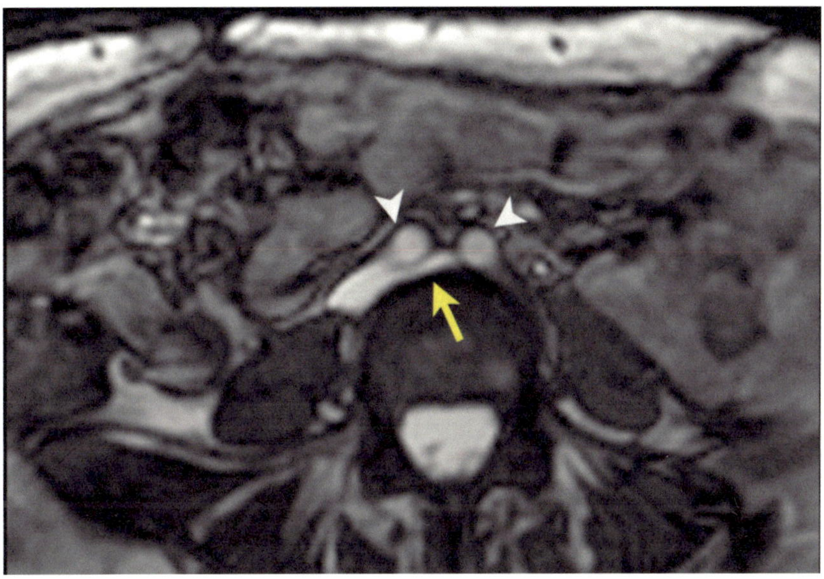

Fig. 2. Bright blood imaging. Balanced steady-state free precession image from an axial cine acquisition demonstrates narrowing of the left common iliac vein (yellow arrow) by the iliac arteries (white arrowheads) and the anterior surface of the L4 vertebral body. This patient had symptoms of May-Thurner syndrome, with recurrent left-sided deep venous thrombosis. Bright blood, or "white blood" imaging yields rapid high-resolution images, although the direction of flowing blood is not discernible.

2.1.3 Time-of-flight imaging of the vessels

Time-of-flight imaging techniques rely on flow-related enhancement to provide signal in the vasculature, and do not require intravascular contrast material. They can be performed via two-dimensional or three-dimensional acquisitions, and depending on the placement of saturation bands, can be tailored to image the arterial or venous system. By acquiring numerous overlapping slices, three-dimensional reformatting can be performed post-hoc to generate more desirable image planes. (Lee 2005)

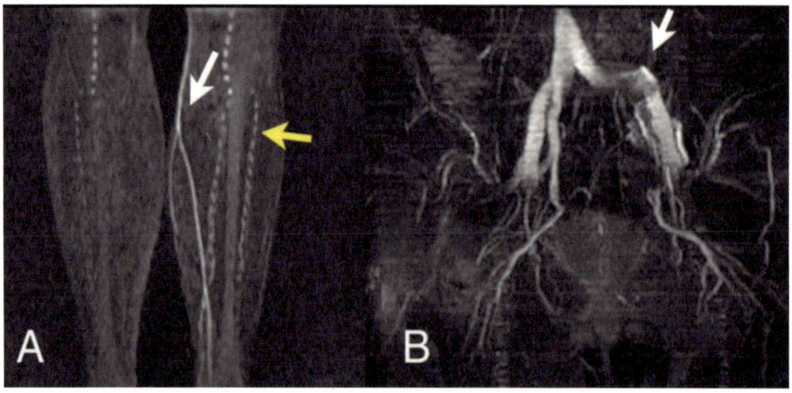

Fig. 3. Time-of-flight versus inflow imaging. Time-of-flight images of the lower legs (A) demonstrate visualization of the left-sided large saphenous veins (white arrow). Note the slab artifacts in the arterial tree which are faintly visualized due to pulsatile flow in the trifurcation vessels (yellow arrow). The patient was suspected of having a more proximal venous obstruction, and inflow techniques with SSFP readout were attempted, yielding a much more robust image of the pelvis (B), which demonstrated compression of the left common iliac vein (white arrow) and numerous small collateral vessels.

2.1.4 Cardiac and respiratory gating

Cardiac and respiratory motion can complicate imaging of the thorax, and even render some acquisitions nondiagnostic. (Boxerman et al. 1998) Certain applications such as cardiac angiography necessitate cardiac gating. This is also particularly true for accurate imaging of the aortic root. (Venkatesh & Ghoshhajra, 2011) Despite this challenge, modern sequences can be rapidly acquired via synchronization to the peripheral plethysmograph or the patient's electrocardiographic leads. Occasionally rapid "real-time" sequences can be used to mitigate cardiac motion without gating, although these images are less frequently acquired due to resolution constraints which render them inferior to gated exams. (Francone et al. 2005) Although breath-held exams are important for much of MRI in and around the thorax, by increasing the number of signal averages the effects of both cardiac and respiratory motion can be mitigated (at the expense of dramatically increased acquisition times). "Navigator-gated" sequences are also available in some cases to acquire bright-blood exams over numerous cardiac and respiratory via a repeated navigator slab which allows rejection of slices acquired during unfavorable respiratory excursions. This technique also dramatically increases acquisition times but again allows free respiration during the exam. (Sakuma et al. 2005)

2.1.5 Inflow imaging

Noncontrast MRA has enjoyed numerous recent technical advances in the form of modified steady-state free precession imaging, which can be tailored for the depiction of flowing

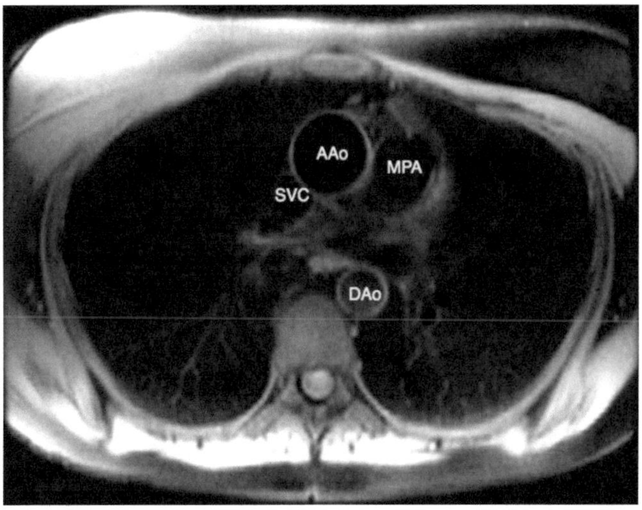

Fig. 4. Cardiac and respiratory gating. Axial black blood imaging of the ascending aorta was obtained with cardiac gating at suspended respiration. This image was obtained with blood suppression to ensure black blood technique, as well as chemical fat suppression. Note the precise depiction of the aortic wall, and motion-free images of the great vessels. The ascending aorta (AAo) has more rapid flow which is perpendicular to the plane of acquisition, and therefore superior blood suppression as compared to the main pulmonary artery (MPA). The superior vena cava (SVC) and descending aorta (DAo) are also well visualized without cardiorespiratory motion artifacts.

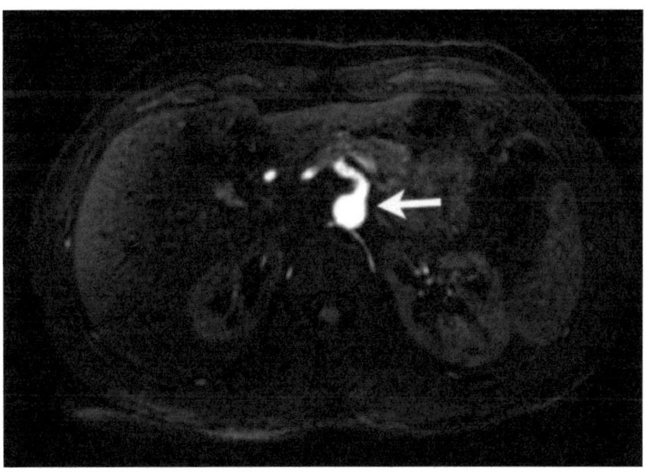

Fig. 5. Inflow imaging. Robust non-contrast MRA can be performed with advanced inflow techniques. In this unenhanced axial source image reconstructed from a three-dimensional steady-state free precession arterial labelled scan the arterial flow in the aorta at its junction with the superior mesenteric artery is well visualized. Note also the opacification of the small intrarenal branches, and relatively low signal from the background tissues.

blood in a rapid acquisition, with or without a directional component. These three-dimensional acquisitions can also be advantageous when the background signal and fat are suppressed, yielding easily reformatted images consisting of moving blood only. These acquisitions can also be synchronized to the peripheral plethysmograph to provide images only in systole or both systole and diastole, thus allowing differentiation from arterial or venous flow in the extremities. (Glockner et al. 2010; Hartung & François, 2011)

3. Contrast-enhanced MRA

Contrast-enhanced MRA can be performed routinely at many centers. These techniques take advantage of the dramatic shortening of T1 relaxation times due to gadolinium's paramagnetic effects. By timing image acquisitions to the arterial or venous phases of circulation (best accomplished via power-injection at a high rate and rapid imaging sequences), the vascular system can be imaged with relative ease. (Lee, 2005) Two recent advances have provided further advantages to contrast-enhanced MRA. In addition to first-pass (arterial) or later phase (venous or equilibrium) timing, extremely rapid images can also be obtained at multiple time points (time-resolved MRA)(Cornfeld & Mojibian, 2009) or images can be obtained very slowly (to improve spatial resolution) when "blood pool" agents are injected, which remain in equilibrium circulation for hours rather than seconds to minutes. (Hansch et al. 2011; Makowski et al. 2011; Hartung & François, 2011)

3.1 Time-resolved MRA

Recent incremental advances in the spatial and temporal resolution of MRA have now allowed multiple rapid successive MRA acquisitions. These techniques have particular relevance when bolus timing is uncertain, or when imaging arteriovenous abnormalities such as arteriovenous malformations or fistulas. (Schanker et al. 2011)

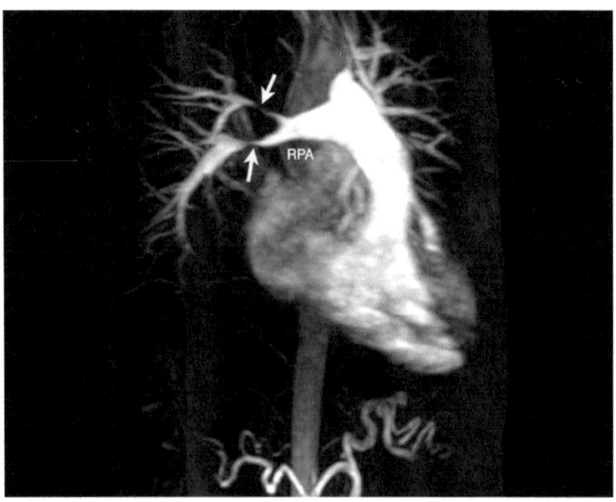

Fig. 6. Time-resolved MRA. Rapid time-resolved MRA is now possible, allowing acquisitions at several time points during the passage of contrast through the circulation. This patient with congenital heart disease suffered from severe stenosis in several branches of the right pulmonary artery (RPA, arrows). Note the relative paucity of contamination by pulmonary venous enhancement on this maximum intensity projection image, which allowed accurate visualization of the pulmonary arterial tree in this pulmonary arterial/early aortic phase image.

4. Image processing techniques for MRA

Most MRA imaging is acquired in coronal or sagittal planes (to decrease acquisition times and phase-wrap artifacts), although some techniques require axial acquisition to allow for flow-related signal acquisitions. A basic tenet of image acquisition is that of isotropic imaging, which then allows later reformatting and volume dataset interpretation. Many images can be reformatted at the scanner or in some cases by a dedicated post-processing laboratory; occasional direct post-processing by the radiologist is preferable. The most common formats are multiplanar reformatting (MPR), maximum-intensity projection reformatting (MIP), and three-dimensional volume-rendered imaging (VR). MPR images allow thin images to be generated from a volume dataset in any plane, whether body-specific planes such as axial images reformatted to coronal or sagittal planes, but also allows curved planar reconstructions along the course of the vessels themselves, which can allow viewing of the entire course of a tortuous vessel in a single image. MIP images are useful for "collapsing" a slab of a volume containing a tortuous vessel into a single image or set of images; this technique is useful but should be reserved as an adjunct to source or MPR images. This is particularly useful for long-axis views, and can be disadvantageous in short-axis reformatting, whereby stenosis can be eliminated from a slab of images. (Wehrschuetz et al. 2004; Regenfus et al. 2003)

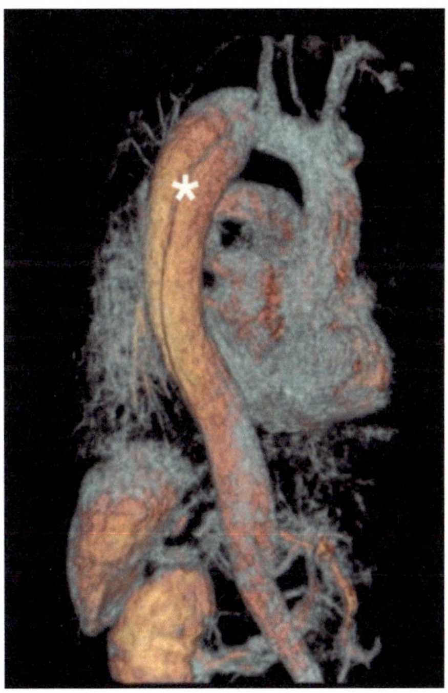

Fig. 7. Volume-rendered imaging. Source images can be reconstructed in several ways. In this case, a three-dimensional volume-rendered image was created to demonstrate the location of an aortic dissection (asterisk). While the appearance can be striking, source and MPR images must be reviewed to ensure that all findings are visualized, since volume rendering only demonstrates the external surface of the enhanced vessels rather than the lumen.

5. Contrast agents for MRA

Gadolinium-based contrast agents have an excellent safety profile, although recent reports of nephrogenic systemic fibrosis (NSF) have dampened enthusiasm and rendered the agents contraindicated in cases of severe renal insufficiency. (Grobner 2005) In patients with normal renal function, these agents have been well tolerated and they enjoy a significantly lower rate of anaphylaxis versus iodinated CT contrast agents. Preserved diagnostic quality with decreased contrast doses can achieved in some cases with the use of high field strength imaging (via improved contrast-to-noise ratios at 3.0 Tesla versus 1.5 Tesla, the two most common field strengths). (Hartung, Grist, and François 2011) All gadolinium-based agents are comprised of paramagnetic chelates that shorten T1 and T2 relaxation times (via disturbance of the spin-lattice and spin-spin interactions). Other contrast agents with various mechanisms of action exist in MRI, but are not utilized routinely for MRA.

5.1 First-pass agents

Traditionally contrast agents in MRA have included gadodiamide, gadobenic acid, gadopentetic acid, and gadoteridol. These are excreted chiefly via renal clearance. Because they are rapidly excreted, timing is critical. (Hartung, Grist, and François 2011)

5.2 Blood pool agents

Recently gadolinium contrast agents have been developed for use in the vascular system, and are advantageous due to slower, predominantly hepatic clearance (gadofosveset).

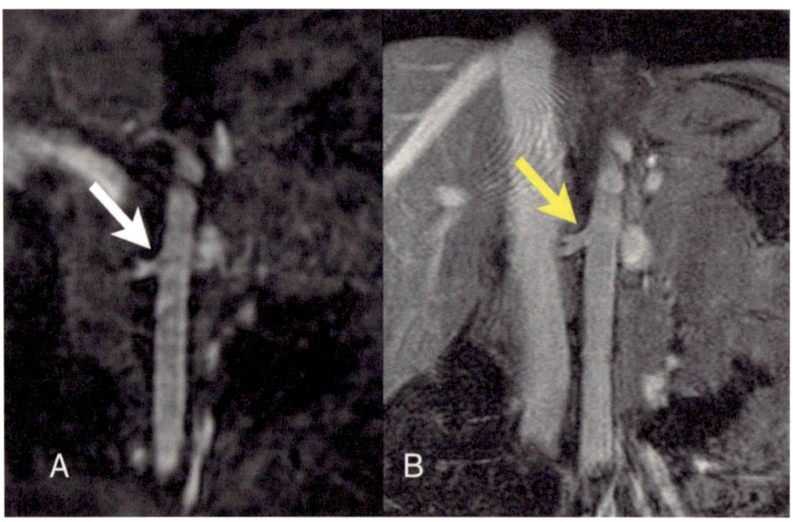

Fig. 8. Dynamic versus blood pool agent imaging. Dynamic first-pass MRA performed with bolus injection of gadofosveset demonstrates pure arterial imaging (A) and equilibrium phase imaging (B). While the arterial phase is not contaminated by venous enhancement, the reduced matrix necessary for rapid imaging (256 x 160 pixels) offers lower spatial resolution than that achieved by equilibrium phase imaging (512 x 224 pixels). The resultant finer voxels offer more robust of small vessel anatomy such as the early branching right renal artery (white arrow in A versus yellow arrow in B).

Although the advantage of such agents is that timing of acquisition is not critical (and can indeed be lengthened in order to image at higher spatial resolutions), by timing a rapid acquisition during the first pass of enhancement a pure arterial phase image set can be obtained prior to equilibrium phase. (Hartung, Grist, and François 2011; Makowski et al. 2011; Hansch et al. 2011)

5.3 Safety and nephrogenic systemic fibrosis

Nephrogenic systemic fibrosis is a disorder that has been associated with renal failure and linked to gadolinium administration. After the disease was identified, dramatic and rapid success in limiting the incidence of new cases was achieved by widespread adoption of guidelines to limit or forgo the use of gadolinium contrast agents in patients with limited renal function as defined by estimated glomerular filtration rates below 60 ml/min/m^2 and 30 ml/min/m^2 respectively. (Kanal et al. 2007)

6. MRA head to toe

Virtually no body part or vascular bed has been untouched by MRA. The pulse sequences, applications, challenges, and utility of MRA varies widely depending on the anatomy imaged. Below is a brief review of the basic MRA applications organized by body system, with a focus on clinical examples of common clinical applications and MRA-specific diagnoses.

6.1 Neurovascular MRA

MRA of the head and neck has rapidly become a mainstay of neuroradiologic practice, in part due to its simultaneous acquisition during MRI of the brain for stroke imaging and workup. The ability to rapidly and accurately screen the cerebrovascular system noninvasively has led to improved stroke care and treatment, and the availability of rapid imaging access defines the capabilities of a stroke center. MRI/MRA access indeed is though to have profound effects upon stroke treatment. Both the arterial and venous systems can be rapidly imaged with and without contrast.

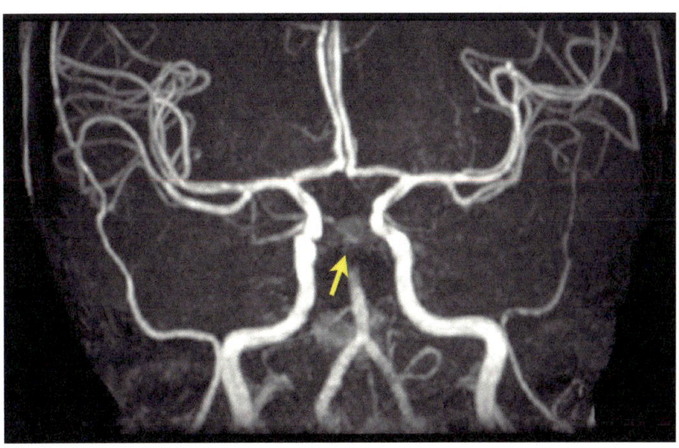

Fig. 9. MRA of the Circle of Willis. Reformatted 3D MRA image demonstrates occlusion of the basilar artery in a patient with acute bilateral central infarcts (aka. "top of the basilar thrombosis syndrome").

6.2 Thoracic MRA

Thoracic MRA plays an increasing role in the workup, diagnosis, and management of aortic disease. While the ease and availability of CT angiography sometimes relegates MRA to a second-line therapy (particularly in the acute setting), MRA of the thoracic vessels is a mainstay of imaging in those patients with a need for repeated longitudinal imaging, such as genetic disorders such as Marfan's syndrome or Loey-Dietz syndrome. The benefits of robust imaging without the need for ionizing radiation (and ability to image without contrast when necessary) makes this test useful for young patients.

6.3 Coronary MRA

Coronary MRA is finally realized as a potential application of cardiac MRI, but its relatively long exam times and inability to depict calcified lesions makes it a second or third choice test for ischemic heart disease. (Lima and Desai 2004) Nonetheless, coronary MRA has demonstrated similar results for the exclusion of significant stenosis to the current noninvasive standard, cardiac-gated CT angiography in small studies. In some applications such as the exclusion of anomalous coronary arteries, MRA has a role, particularly in younger population in whom atherosclerotic stenosis is unlikely.

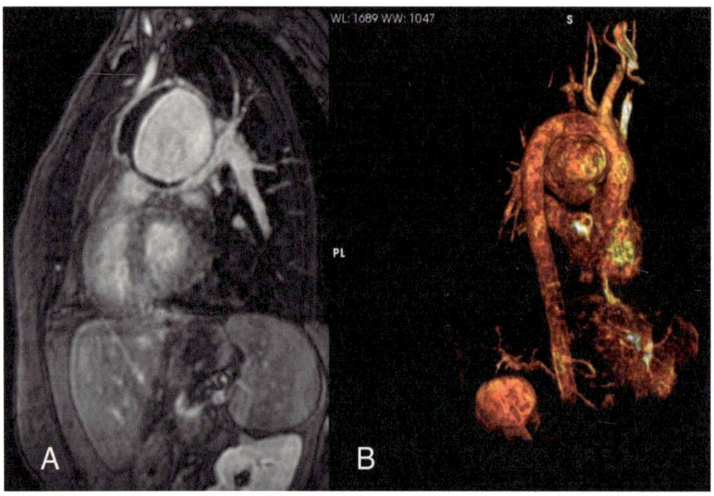

Fig. 10. MRA of the aortic arch. Sagittal MIP (A) and 3D volume-rendered (B) images of the thoracic aortic arch demonstrate a large, saccular pseudoaneurysm in a patient whom developed a myocotic aneurysm due to immunosuppression by chemotherapy.

6.4 Abdominopelvic MRA

MRI/MRA is increasingly useful in many body imaging applications. The technique is useful for the workup of vascular hepatic lesions, and is robust for the imaging of large vessels such as abdominal aortic aneurysms. Although artifacts can limit the utility for imaging small vessels, MRA is often useful in young patients or patients whom are able to breath-hold and comply with the exam. In conjunction with anatomic imaging, MRA can be invaluable in certain workups, such as preoperative planning for uterine artery embolization.

6.5 Peripheral MRA

Limb ischemia is often a chronic disease requiring intense longitudinal follow-up, and imaging can play a central role. The utility of MRA in the management of peripheral vascular disease can be large, because the technique can obviate invasive arteriography and in many cases lead to shorter exam times when invasive angiography is deemed necessary. MRA, and in particular dynamic MRA, can be useful in the workup of more rare lesions such as vascular malformations.

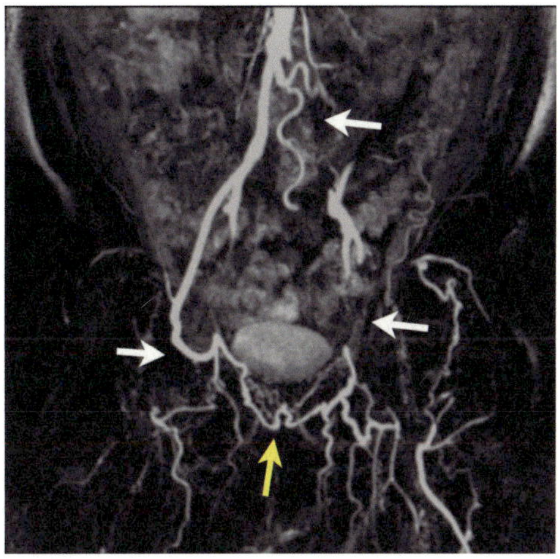

Fig. 11. MRA of the aortoiliac vessels. Coronal MIP image from a contrast-enhanced MRA demonstrates multiple occlusions (white arrows) and right-to-left collaterals (yellow arrow) in a patient with severe atherosclerotic disease.

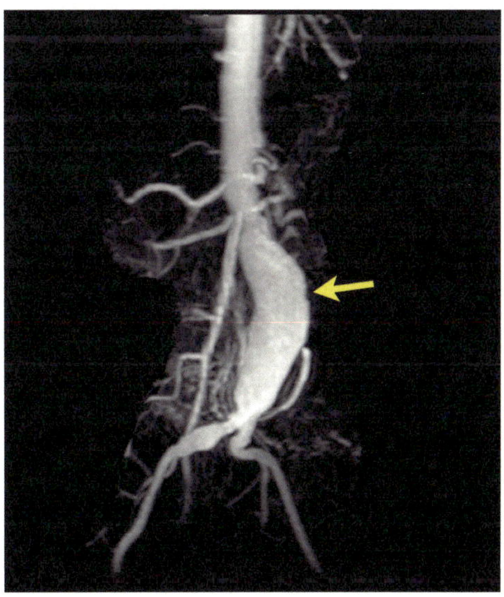

Fig. 12. MRA for abdominal aortic aneurysm. Oblique coronal MIP image from a contrast-enhanced MRA demonstrates a saccular infrarenal aortic aneurysm. MRA is particularly useful in patients whom need repeated imaging for longitudinal followup.

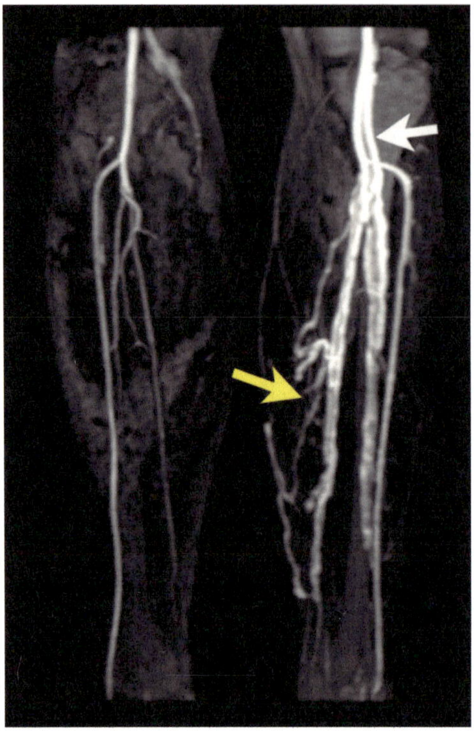

Fig. 13. MRA of the lower extremities. Coronal MIP image from a contrast-enhanced MRA demonstrates early filling of left-sided veins in a patient with claudication due to congenital arteriovenous malformations.

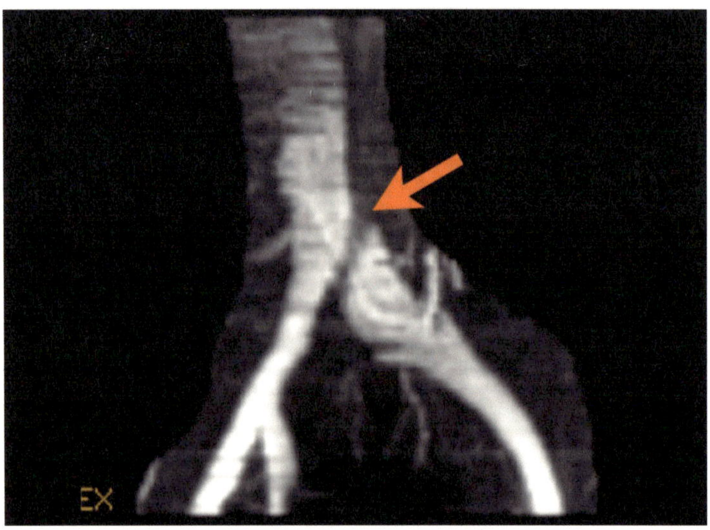

Fig. 14. MR venography of the pelvic veins. Reformatted image from a noncontrast inflow-based acquisition of the pelvic veins demonstrates compression of the left common iliac vein by the right common iliac artery in a patient with left to right venous collaterals and chronic left-sided deep venous thrombosis due to May-Thurner syndrome.

6.6 MR venography

In addition to the more common use of MRA for the arterial system, numerous venous beds can be reliably imaged with MRA. In the neurovascular system, the importance of venous thrombosis is now widely recognized, and in the pelvic circulation MRA plays a key role due to the ability to acquire multiple phases of imaging and image external compression on the veins in cases of May-Thurner syndrome. Although initial enthusiasm for MRA of the pulmonary arteries was high, trials have shown difficulties with MRA of thromboembolic disease in the chest and a high rate of nondiagnostic examinations. (Stein et al. 2008)

7. MRA artifacts

While the power and reach of MRA is impressive, the technique is not without difficulties. Artifacts can confound this robust technique, and each sequence carries with it its own technical pitfalls. The lack of standard appearances across multiple sequences, planes, and phases of contrast enhancement makes the task of the radiologist even more challenging. A vigilant eye and sceptical mind are essential. A rule of thumb in vascular imaging is to assume that all findings are artifactual until proven otherwise; if the presence of counfounding artifacts can be systematically excluded, then one can presume the findings are indeed real.

7.1 Motion artifacts

MRA sequences can be time-consuming, and the presence of motion artifact can be encountered as patients are unable to comply with a long acquisition (Figure 15), or due to normal cardiac or respiratory motion (Figure 16)

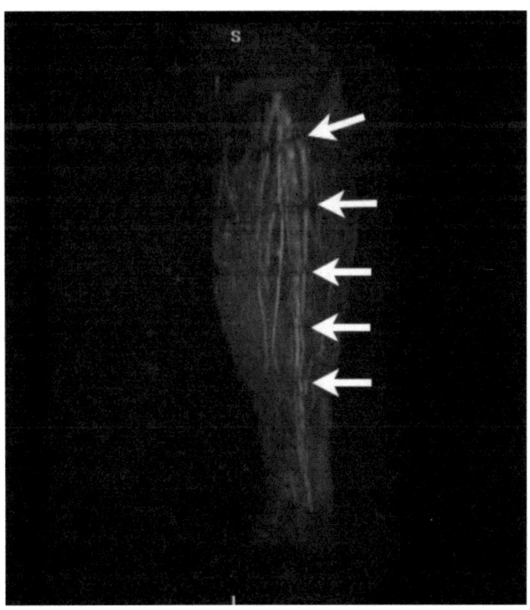

Fig. 15. Time-of-flight MRA of the lower extremity. Reformatted image from a noncontrast time-of-flight sequence obtained as multiple axial acquisitions (and later reformatted into this coronal view) demonstrates numerous banding artifacts (white arrows) which were introduced by patient motion during the exam.

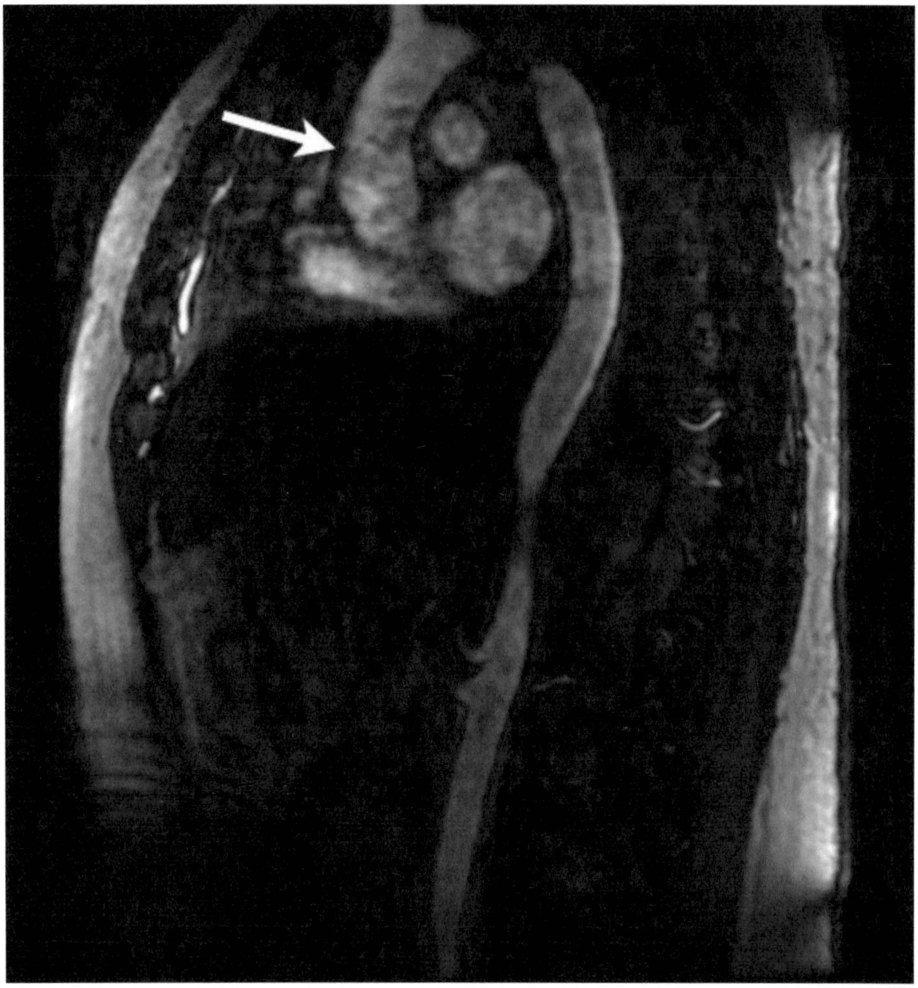

Fig. 16. Contrast MRA of the Aortic Arch. Sagittal reformatted image from a bolus contrast-enhanced MRA performed to exclude aortic dissection shows motion artifact causing irregularity of the ascending thoracic aorta (white arrow). This is due to cardiac pulsation during acquisition.

7.2 Timing artifacts

MRA sequences performed during bolus contrast enhancement must be performed with proper timing in order to image the target vascular bed at the appropriate time. Improper timing can make interpretation difficult or impossible (Figure 17).

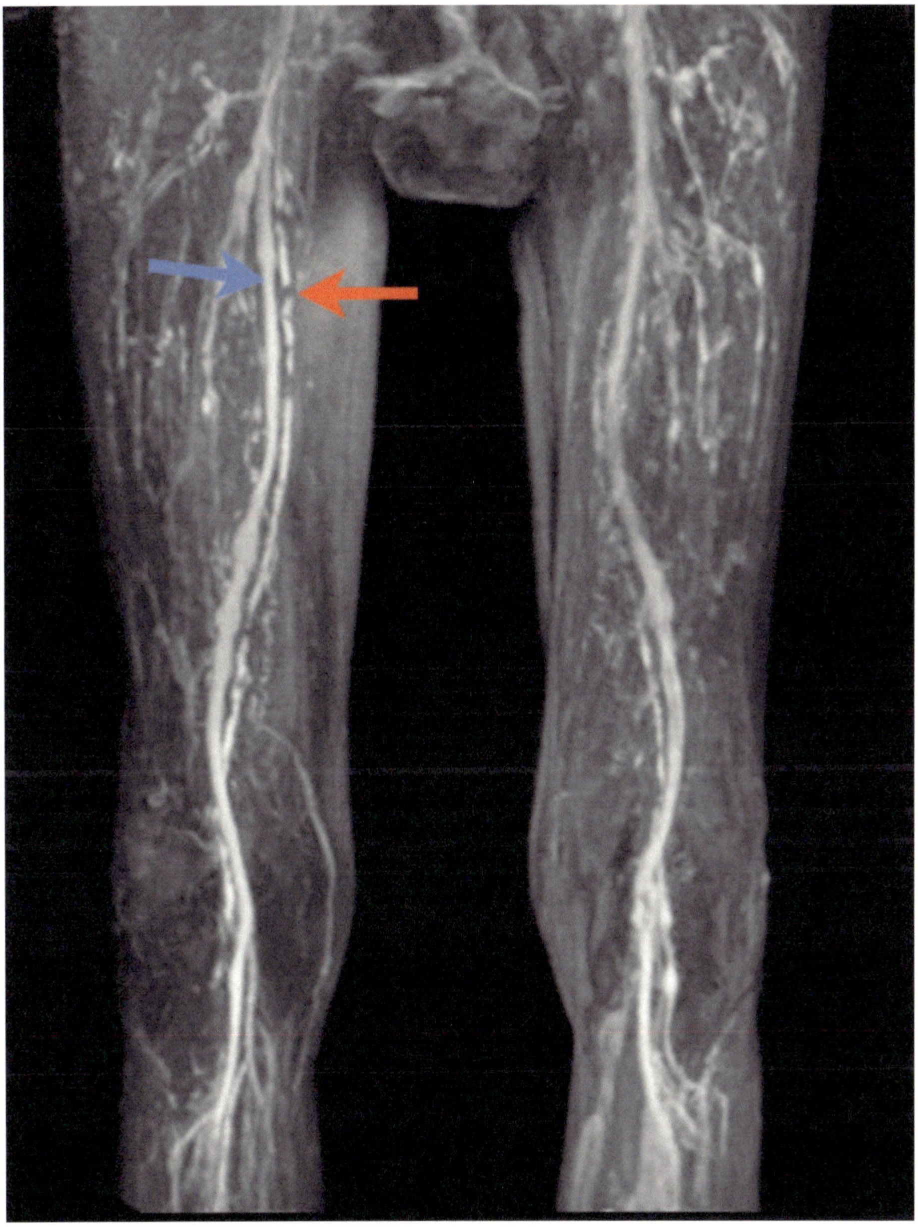

Fig. 17. Suboptimal bolus timing. Coronal reformatted image from a bolus contrast-enhanced MRA performed to exclude stenosis of the lower extremity arteries is confounded by venous contamination (blue arrow), which makes the highly diseased arterial system (red arrow) difficult to visualize. This was in part due to extremely poor cardiac function.

7.3 Difficult body habitus and positioning

MRI can be a challenge due to issues with large patients, whom may not fit into the bore of the magnet, or may be so large as to cause phase wrap artifacts affecting the vessel of interest (Figure 18).

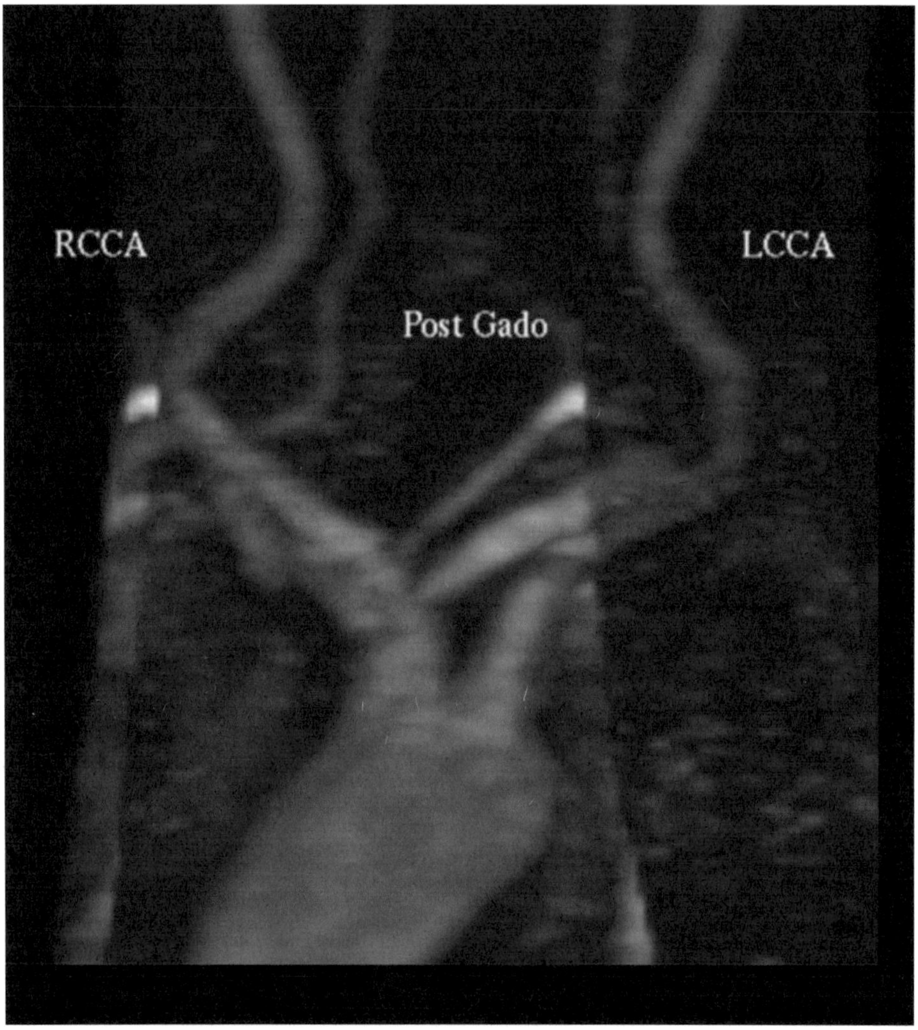

Fig. 18. Phase wrap artifact. This large patient's body habitus resulted in phase wrap of the right shoulder over the left common carotid artery; poor signal to noise ratio is therefore made worse at the site of the wrap artifact.

7.4 Metallic artifacts

MRI can also be a limited due to the radiofrequency shielding effects of metal in the body, particularly within stents (Figures 19 and 20).

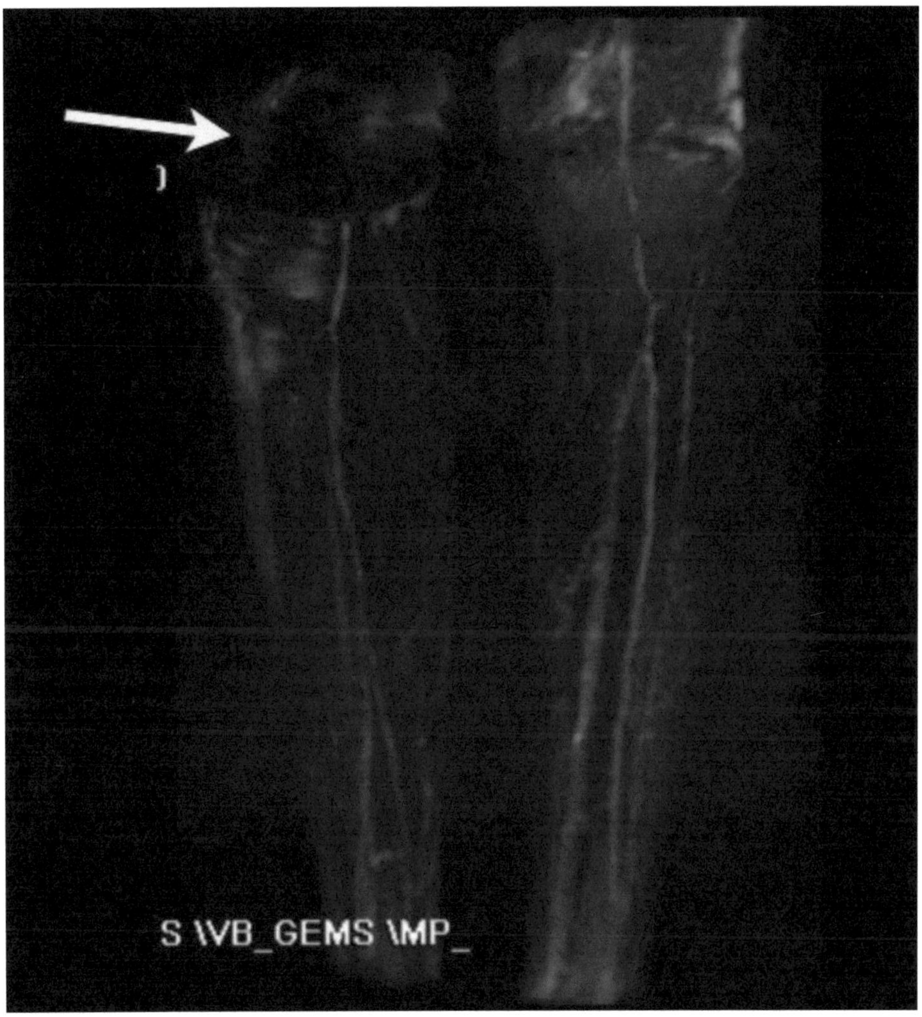

Fig. 19. Metallic implant artifact (magnetic susceptibility artifact). This patient's right knee prosthesis caused apparent occlusion (white arrow) of the right popliteal artery (which was actually widely patent).

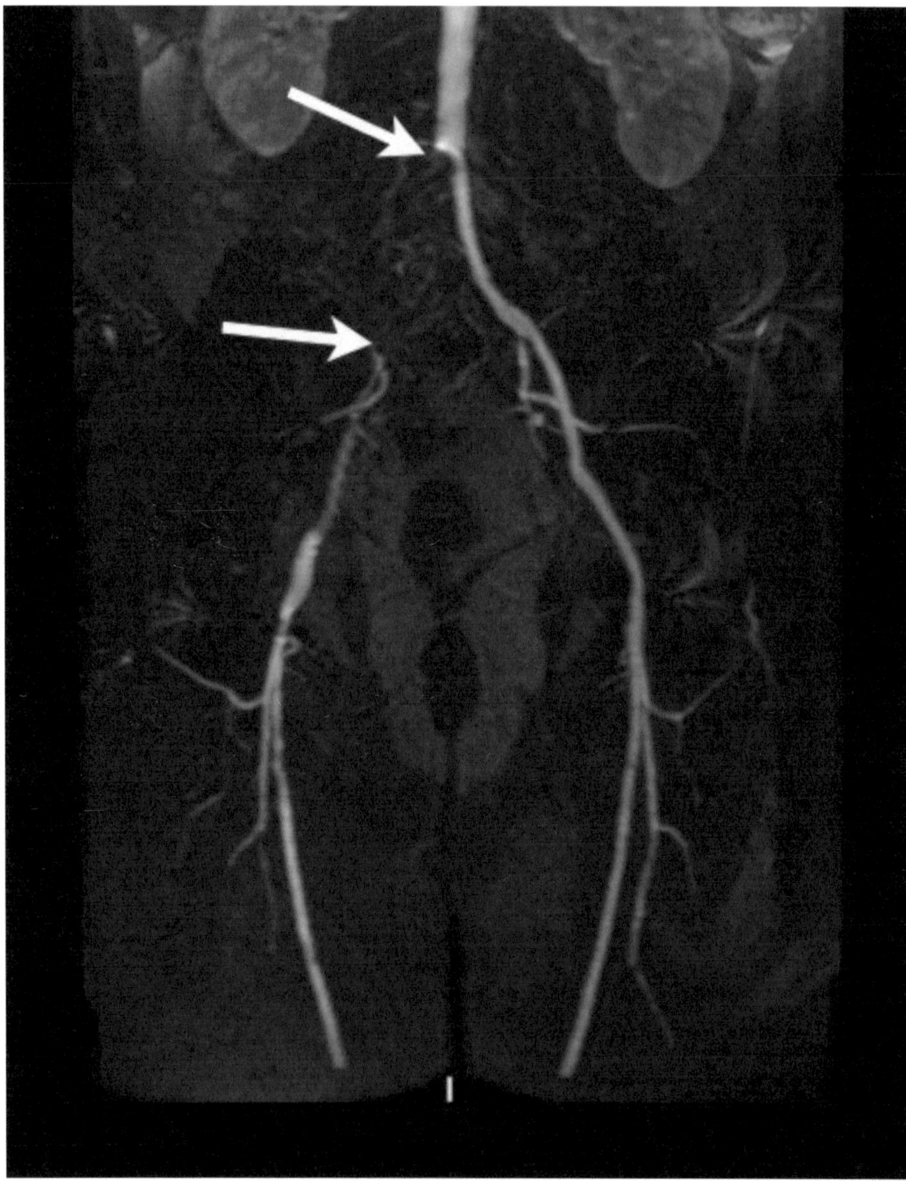

Fig. 20. Radiofrequency shielding artifact (magnetic susceptibility artifact). This patient's right common iliac stent created the appearance of arterial occlusion (white arrow); note the lack of collaterals and dephasing artifact (upper arrow) which are clues to the artifactual nature of the findings.

8. Conclusion

Magnetic resonance angiography is increasingly a part of the workup of vascular disease throughout the body, and is a central part of imaging for several diseases. The impact of MRA will continue in parallel to the development of newer and more robust pulse sequences.

9. Acknowledgment

The authors wish to thank the technologist, staff, and referring physicians of The Massachusetts General Hospital for their continued dedication to excellence in the care of patients and the support of the field of magnetic resonance imaging.

10. References

Boxerman, J L, T J Mosher, E R McVeigh, E Atalar, J A Lima, and D A Bluemke. 1998. "Advanced MR imaging techniques for evaluation of the heart and great vessels." *Radiographics : a review publication of the Radiological Society of North America, Inc* 18 (3): 543–564.

Cornfeld, D, and H Mojibian. 2009. "Clinical Uses of Time-Resolved Imaging in the Body and Peripheral Vascular System." *American Journal of Roentgenology* 193 (6) (November 20): W546–W557. doi:10.2214/AJR.09.2826.

Francone, Marco, Steven Dymarkowski, Maria Kalantzi, and Jan Bogaert. 2005. "Real-time cine MRI of ventricular septal motion: a novel approach to assess ventricular coupling." *Journal of magnetic resonance imaging : JMRI* 21 (3) (March 1): 305–309. doi:10.1002/jmri.20259.

Glockner, James F, Naoki Takahashi, Akira Kawashima, David A Woodrum, David W Stanley, Naoyuki Takei, Mitsuharu Miyoshi, and Wei Sun. 2010. "Non-contrast renal artery MRA using an inflow inversion recovery steady state free precession technique (Inhance): comparison with 3D contrast-enhanced MRA.." *Journal of magnetic resonance imaging : JMRI* 31 (6) (June): 1411–1418. doi:10.1002/jmri.22194.

Grobner, T. 2005. "Gadolinium - a specific trigger for the development of nephrogenic fibrosing dermopathy and nephrogenic systemic fibrosis?." *Nephrology Dialysis Transplantation* 21 (4) (December 19): 1104–1108. doi:10.1093/ndt/gfk062.

Hansch, Andreas, Stefan Betge, Gunther Poehlmann, Steffi Neumann, Pascal Baltzer, Alexander Pfeil, Matthias Waginger, et al. 2011. "Combined magnetic resonance imaging of deep venous thrombosis and pulmonary arteries after a single injection of a blood pool contrast agent." *European Radiology* 21 (2) (February 1): 318–325. doi:10.1007/s00330-010-1918-0.

Hartung, Michael P, Thomas M Grist, and Christopher J François. 2011. "Magnetic resonance angiography: current status and future directions.." *J Cardiovasc Magn Reson* 13: 19. doi:10.1186/1532-429X-13-19.

Kanal, E, A J Barkovich, C Bell, J P Borgstede, W G Bradley, J W Froelich, T Gilk, et al. 2007. "ACR Guidance Document for Safe MR Practices: 2007." *American Journal of Roentgenology* 188 (6) (June 1): 1447–1474. doi:10.2214/AJR.06.1616.

Lee, Vivian S. 2005. *Cardiovascular MR Imaging: Physical Principles to Practical Protocols.* 1st ed. Lippincott Williams & Wilkins, December 14.

Lima, João A C, and Milind Y Desai. 2004. "Cardiovascular magnetic resonance imaging: current and emerging applications." *Journal of the American College of Cardiology* 44 (6) (September 15): 1164–1171. doi:10.1016/j.jacc.2004.06.033.

Macovski, Albert. 2009. "MRI: a charmed past and an exciting future.." *Journal of magnetic resonance imaging : JMRI* 30 (5) (November): 919–923. doi:10.1002/jmri.21962.

Makowski, Marcus R, Andrea J Wiethoff, Sergio Uribe, Victoria Parish, René M Botnar, Aaron Bell, Christoph Kiesewetter, et al. 2011. "Congenital Heart Disease: Cardiovascular MR Imaging by Using an Intravascular Blood Pool Contrast Agent.." *Radiology* 260 (3) (September): 680–688. doi:10.1148/radiol.11102327.

Nath, H. 2006. "The Legacy of 'Visualization of the Chambers of the Heart, the Pulmonary Circulation, and the Great Blood Vessels in Man'." *American Journal of Roentgenology* 186 (6) (June 1): 1489–1490. doi:10.2214/AJR.05.1941.

Regenfus, M., D. Ropers, S Achenbach, C. Schlundt, W. Kessler, G Laub, W. Moshage, and W. G. Daniel. 2003. "Diagnostic value of maximum intensity projections versus source images for assessment of contrast-enhanced three-dimensional breath-hold magnetic resonance coronary angiography." *Investigative radiology* 38 (4). Invest Radiol (April): 200–206. doi:10.1097/01.RLI.0000057030.71459.7F.

Sakuma, Hajime, Yasutaka Ichikawa, Naohisa Suzawa, Tadanori Hirano, Katsutoshi Makino, Nozomu Koyama, Marc Van Cauteren, and Kan Takeda. 2005. "Assessment of coronary arteries with total study time of less than 30 minutes by using whole-heart coronary MR angiography." *Radiology* 237 (1) (October 1): 316–321. doi:10.1148/radiol.2371040830.

Saloner, D. 1995. "The AAPM/RSNA physics tutorial for residents. An introduction to MR angiography.." *Radiographics : a review publication of the Radiological Society of North America, Inc* 15 (2) (March): 453–465.

Schanker, Benjamin D, Brian P Walcott, Brian V Nahed, Christopher S Ogilvy, Andrew J M Kiruluta, James D Rabinov, and William A Copen. 2011. "Time-resolved contrast-enhanced magnetic resonance angiography in the investigation of suspected intracranial dural arteriovenous fistula.." *Journal of clinical neuroscience : official journal of the Neurosurgical Society of Australasia* 18 (6) (June): 837–839. doi:10.1016/j.jocn.2010.12.003.

Seldinger, S I. 1953. "Catheter replacement of the needle in percutaneous arteriography; a new technique.." *Acta radiologica* 39 (5) (May): 368–376.

Stein, Paul D, Alexander Gottschalk, H Dirk Sostman, Thomas L Chenevert, Sarah E Fowler, Lawrence R Goodman, Charles A Hales, et al. 2008. "Methods of Prospective Investigation of Pulmonary Embolism Diagnosis III (PIOPED III)." *Seminars in nuclear medicine* 38 (6) (November 1): 462–470. doi:10.1053/j.semnuclmed.2008.06.003.

Venkatesh, Vikram, Daniel Verdini, and Brian Ghoshhajra MD MBA. 2011. "Normal Magnetic Resonance Imaging of the Thorax." *Magnetic resonance imaging clinics of North America* (June). doi:10.1016/j.mric.2011.05.014.

Wehrschuetz, M, M Aschauer, H Portugaller, A Stix, E Wehrschuetz-Sigl, K Hausegger, and F Ebner. 2004. "Review of source images is necessary for the evaluation of gadolinium-enhanced MR angiography for renal artery stenosis.." *Cardiovascular and interventional radiology* 27 (5) (August): 441–446. doi:10.1007/s00270-004-0047-z.

2

MR Angiography and Development: Review of Clinical Applications

Amit Mehndiratta[1], Michael V. Knopp[2] and Fredrik L. Giesel[1]
[1]University of Heidelberg,
[2]Ohio State University, Ohio,
[1]Germany
[2]USA

1. Introduction

Contrast-enhanced Magnetic Resonance Angiography (CR-MRA) is remarkable technique to image the vascular system from head to toe in diagnostic imaging armoury. Computed tomography is still an adequate imaging method of choice in few applications such as in follow-up studies in neuro-vascular pathologies, even then MRA is getting an equal share with tremendous improvements in spatial and temporal resolution. Current clinical indications for MRA of the supra-aortic vessels in head and neck include evaluation of steno-occlusive disease, assessment of AV-malformations in cerebral vessels, aneurysms, atherosclerotic disease and dissections. Moreover, as with other imaging applications, limiting contrast dose is a major issue, particularly with the increased risk of development of Nephrogenic Systemic Fibrosis (NSF) with higher doses of contrast agent [1] [2]. Therefore, contrast agents with higher relaxivity or higher concentration (1M), for which lower doses may be used, are beneficial for dynamic MRA studies.

The critical advantages of Gd-contrast agent for MRA of the vessels are: increased signal-to-noise ratio and greater vessel conspicuity. In this chapter we will discuss in detail the benefits and limitations of currently available gadolinium contrast agents for MRA with respect to its clinical indications. We will focus on gadofosveset [3;4] as well, it is relatively a new contrast available in clinical applications and would be nice to compare its benefits and limitations with other Gadolinium contrast agents which have been used for long in clinical environment.

2. Conventional technique of magnetic resonance imaging angiography

MR imaging depends on the relaxation times (T1, T2 and T2*) and proton density in the tissue of interest. MRI is very sensitive to flow and motions originating during image acquisition. The motions induced by flow can be responsible for number of artefacts which can drastically impair the diagnostic image value but on other hand sometime these flow effects are of vital interest to image the vascular anatomy. The MRA can be classified to time of flight (TOF) and phase contrast MRA [5]. In TOF MRA the blood flow is assumed to be perpendicular to the plane of acquisition. For repetition time (TR) shorter than the longitudinal T1 relaxation of the stationary proton spins in the imaging slice, the signal will be reduced due to partial saturation effect (saturating RF pulse). Inflow blood in the vessel will move the spins from outside of the slice into the imaging plane; these spins have not been subjected to the spatially selective RF pulse. These unsaturated spins upon entering the slice will produce a much stronger signal than stationary spins assuming the gradient echo sequence is applied. This effect is called "entry slice phenomenon" or "inflow enhancement" or "flow related enhancement". The amount of inflow enhancement will depend on various factors like tissue properties (T1), sequence parameters (flip angle and TR) and geometrical parameters (slice thickness, orientation and flow velocity). TOF is based on fundamental principle that any vessels segment can be imaged by cutting through the vessel perpendicular to the flow direction [5]. With this repetitive method applied at each slice a complete three dimensional data of vascular tree can be acquired. Various multiple 3D reformatting algorithms are available with the post processing unit (Maximum Intensity Projection) which can help radiologist visualise the complex vascular anatomy with appropriate precision [5]. The image acquisition can be 2D or 3D (as other MRI sequences). Both techniques are currently used in clinic with specific applications. The 2D techniques offers a higher vessels/background contrast hence can be used in slow flow zone but 3D method is limited to fast flow situations. Another aspect of choice among two is the spatial resolution. In 2D technique the inplane resolution depends on the FOV and matrix size resulting in an anisotropic volume where slice thickness is usually higher than inplane resolution. Whereas the isotropic resolution can be achieved with 3D techniques up to sub-millimetre scale, in addition offers a better signal to noise ratio due to averaging effect of the phase encoding in slab direction.

Phase contrast Angiography: This class of MRA is based on the changes in the phase of transverse magnetization [5]. The phase shifts occur when the spins move along a magnetic field gradient. The flow induced phase shift has a linear relationship with the moving velocity. Hence flow induced phase shift can be used for flow quantification. The phase contrast MRA is acquired as two data sets with different flow sensitivity. The first data (S1) is acquired with flow compensation (no flow sensitivity), whereas the second (S2) is acquired with flow sensitivity. The amount of sensitivity is controlled by gradient strength. The length of the complex difference between S1 and S2 is dependent on the phase shift. An image with signal intensity of difference represents the velocity of the spins within the field of view.

3. Contrast enhanced MRA

The paramagnetic extracellular contrast agent (Gd chelates) increases the blood signal by shortening the T1 relaxation time of the blood. Thus the blood produces the highest signal compared to tissue; hence vessel lumen can be demarcated with maximum intensity projections. There are various Gd- contrast agents available with different properties and relaxivities (table 1) [6-8]. Each one has different relaxivity at different field strength (table 2) [6-9] which is very important to know for practical applications. The details of various gadolinium contrast agent [10;11] properties are beyond the scope of this chapter, we will focus on the application of these contrast agents in various clinical conditions.

4. Magnetic resonance angiography of head and neck

The information provided by magnetic resonance imaging (MRI) in evaluation of brain lesions is critical for accurate diagnosis, therapeutic intervention and prognosis [12]. Contrast enhanced MR neuroimaging using gadolinium (Gd) contrast agents depicts blood-

Agent	Trade name	Manufacturer	Concentration (mol/l)	Protein-binding	r1*	r2*
Gadobenate dimeglumine	MultiHance®	Bracco Diagnostics	0.5	Weak	9.7–10.8	12.2–12.5
Gadodiamide	Omniscan™	GE Healthcare	0.5	None	4.8	5.1
Gadopentetate dimeglumine	Magnevist®	Bayer Schering Pharma AG	0.5	None	4.9–5.0	5.4–6.3
Gadoteridol	ProHance®	Bracco Diagnostics	0.5	None	4.6	5.3
Gadoversetamide	OptiMARK®	Mallinckrodt	0.5	None	NA	NA
Gadoterate meglumine	Dotarem®	Guerbet	0.5	None	4.3	5.0
Gadobutrol	Gadovist®	Bayer Schering Pharma AG	1.0	None	5.6 [41]	NA
Gadofosveset	Vasovist®	Bayer Schering Pharma AG	0.25	Strong	33.4 to 45.7 mM-1 s-1 (0.47 T)	NA

*Measured at 0.47 T in human serum or plasma

Table 1. Gadolinium contrast agents used in MR Imaging [6-8].

		Gd-BOPTA		Gd-DTPA	
Field strength	Source	r1 ($l/mmol^{-1}\cdot s^{-1}$)	r2 ($l/mmol^{-1}\cdot s^{-1}$)	r1 ($l/mmol^{-1}\cdot s^{-1}$)	r2 ($l/mmol^{-1}\cdot s^{-1}$)
0.2 T	Pintaske[a]	10.9	18.9	5.7	9.2
0.47 T	de Haën[b]	9.7	12.5	4.9[d]	6.3[d]
	Rohrer[c]	9.2	12.9	3.8	4.1
1.5 T	Pintaske[a]	7.9	18.9	3.9	5.3
	Rohrer[c]	6.3	8.7	4.1	4.6
3.0 T	Pintaske[a]	5.9	17.5	3.9	5.2
	Rohrer[c]	5.5	11.0	3.7	5.2

Gd-BOPTA=gadobenate dimeglumine; Gd-DTPA=gadopentetate dimeglumine

(a) In human plasma at 37°C

(b) In heparinised human plasma at 39°C

(c) In bovine plasma at 40°C

(d) In heparinised human plasma

Table 2. Relaxivities of Gadobenate dimeglumine and gadopentetate dimeglumine at varying magnetic field strengths [6-9].

brain barrier disruption, thereby demonstrating the location and extent of the disease by depicting the increased EES contrast concentration in these areas. Simple contrast-enhanced morphologic imaging, however, is limited in accurately predicting tumor aggressiveness [13]. Adding dynamic contrast-enhanced and perfusion weighted imaging [14] can solve this problem by providing physiological information (hemodynamic and neoangiogenic status) in addition to pure lesion morphology [15-17].

Most of available Gd-contrast agents differ in their T1 and T2 relaxivities, but have a comparable tissue enhancing properties. The exceptions are gadobenate, gadoxetate and gadofosveset [4], all of which have transient protein binding capability that is responsible for up to twice (and more) the R1 and R2 relaxivity as compared to the other agents at all magnetic field strengths [8] [18;19]. In this section, we summarize the current clinical applications of gadolinium contrast agents in neuroimaging.

Bueltmann et.al [20] conducted a study comparing equal single doses of gadobenate dimeglumine and gadopentetate dimeglumine for CE-MRA of the supra-aortic vessels at 3T in 12 healthy volunteers. Qualitative image analysis revealed significantly higher (p=0.031) values in all the examinations with a gadobenate dimeglumine [7;21]. The overall score for vessel delineation was also significantly (p=0.005) higher and in general a significant (p≤0.026) preference for gadobenate dimeglumine was noted as well as specifically for assessments of the extracranial arteries, Circle of Willis and vessels distal to the Circle of Willis. In addition, gadobenate dimeglumine use demonstrated significantly (p≤0.021) greater rCNR (relative contrast to noise ratio) for the internal carotid, middle cerebral and basilar arteries [22].

The 1M formulation of gadobutrol permits a 50% reduction in the bolus injection volume, thus it has been hypothesised that this reduced volume along with a faster injection rate would facilitate a sharper peak in the contrast bolus, therefore a better first-pass MRA signal [23;24]. However, the results from few clinical studies have been in disagreement with the hypothesis. In a small intraindividual study (N=12); patients received a single dose of 1M gadobutrol and a double dose of 0.5M gadopentetate dimeglumine, a significantly higher SNR and CNR, and better delineation of arterial morphology, was observed with the 1M agent [25;26]. However, in another volunteer study, 5 healthy volunteers underwent 4 consecutive MRA examinations with: a single dose of 1M gadobutrol, a single dose of 1M gadobutrol diluted to twice the volume, and single doses of gadopentetate dimeglumine and gadobenate dimeglumine for which the volume and flow rate were doubled to match the diluted gadobutrol volume and concentration. Quantitatively, the SNR and CNR for gadobenate dimeglumine and both standard and diluted forms of gadobutrol were significantly ($p<0.02$) higher than gadopentetate dimeglumine [27;28], yet no significant difference between either form of gadobutrol and gadobenate dimeglumine was reported [12]. Overall, it seems that 1M gadobutrol may or may not be advantageous for MRA of supra aortic vessels, depending on the vascular territory being examined but it has never demonstrated benefit beyond the higher relaxivity agents for CE-MRA [20;27-29]. But it has been proved that gadobutrol is benefiticial in brain perfusion imaging than gadopentetate dimeglumine (Figure 1 courtesy) [23].

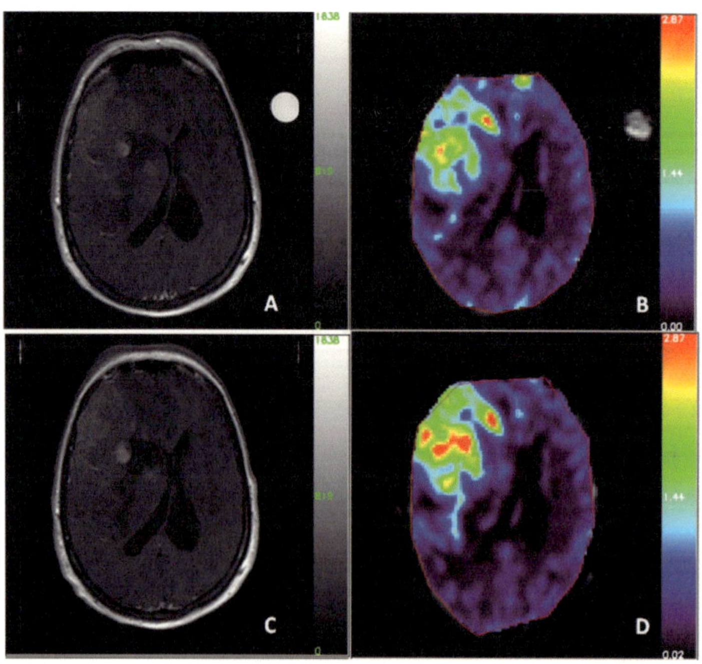

Fig. 1. Intraaxial tumor: T1-weighted image (A) with Gd-DTPA showing a brain tumor in the frontal lobe of the right hemisphere; maximum concentration color map for perfusion-weighted image with Gd-DTPA (B). T1-weighted image with gadobutrol (C); maximum concentration color map for perfusion-weighted image with gadobutrol (D).

Blood pool agents such as gadofosveset (Vasovist®) remain in the circulation for an extended time and thus might be potentially useful for imaging of the vasculature [8]. Benefits of steady state MRA imaging of the head and neck with blood pool agents are anticipated because of its high relaxivity and the extended imaging time associated with its use. CE-MRA with gadofosveset, the only blood pool agent approved for use, has demonstrated improvements in sensitivity, specificity and accuracy compared with non-contrast time-of-flight MRA. However, the benefit of gadofosveset compared with other Gd-contrast agents has been more difficult to establish [4]. Studies have shown that gadofosveset is superior to gadoterate meglumine (Dotarem®) and gadopentetate dimeglumine for MRA of the hand and whole body [3], respectively. While for MRA of the peripheral arteries, gadobenate dimeglumine significantly more specific ($p<0.0001$) and gadofosveset was found to be significantly more sensitive ($p=0.011$) [3].

5. Magnetic resonance angiography of pulmonary vessels

Selective visualization of the pulmonary arteries and veins in high spatial resolution has been the domain of conventional digital subtraction angiography. Drawbacks of the technique were its invasiveness, the use of nephrotoxic contrast media, and long exposure to ionizing radiation. The traditional MRA techniques (including time-of-flight and phase-contrast angiography), with long acquisition times, were substantially limited by motion artifacts, inplane saturation, and intravoxel dephasing. In particular, this affected visualization of small pulmonary vessel details.

With the introduction of three-dimensional gadolinium-enhanced MRA (3D-Gd-MRA), the limitations of non-enhanced MRA were overcome. The high-resolution pulmonary angiograms could be acquired in a single breath hold without use of nephrotoxic contrast media and radiation exposure [30;31]. CE-MRA has already been established as a safe and reliable technique for the detection of pulmonary embolism. However, overlay of arteries and veins in single-phase acquisitions with scan times of over 20 seconds affects the diagnostic reliability, particularly if assessed by the maximum intensity projection (MIP) algorithm. Several clinical scenarios require a dedicated selective assessment of pulmonary arteries and veins. In 30% of young patients with cerebrovascular accident (CVA), no underlying etiology is found. In these patients, pulmonary venous thrombosis has been suspected as the source of emboli, which was confirmed by autopsy later in some cases [32-34]. For accurate surgical pre-planning in patients with pulmonary arterio-venous malformations or bronchial carcinoma, a detailed analysis of the arterial and venous pulmonary vasculature is mandatory. Multiphase angiography with very short acquisition times in each of the single time-resolved phases has produced pure arterio- and venograms of the lungs at the cost of substantially lower spatial resolution and anatomic coverage [35].

The image quality of 3D-Gd-MRA has remarkably improved within the last few years up to a point at which vascular pathologies are detected with accuracy similar to that by the conventional digital subtraction angiography [36]. This is primary possible by the faster sequences, which allow higher resolution scans within a single breath-hold acquisition. In addition, optimized strategies for bolus timing and acquisition during maximum arterial gadolinium concentrations have substantially contributed to consistently high image quality. However, the problem remained of imaging structures separately with rapid sequential enhancement. This includes imaging of pulmonary arteries without overlay of veins or renal arteries without overlay of renal parenchyma [37]. It is expected to improve with faster acquisition sequences and further improvement in MRA technology.

In short we can say that the diagnostic workup of many pulmonary diseases has improved tremendously by the non-invasive, safe technique of CE-MRA. Surgical planning could benefit from the selective 3D visualization of arteries and veins compressed or invaded by centrally growing tumors. The different components of arteriovenous malformations including feeding and draining vessels could be selectively visualized, and the rate of contrast fill-in and transit could be assessed. This also includes monitoring of the lesion after interventional embolization. Selective venograms are particularly useful to assess the pulmonary venous system for thrombi.

6. Magnetic resonance angiography of heart and coronary arteries

Magnetic Resonance Angiography is the most attractive of angiography procedures for Coronary arteries because of its widespread clinical availability and the absence of ionizing radiations. Kim et al [38] performed a multicentre trial in which coronary magnetic resonance angiography revealed left main or three-vessel disease with a sensitivity of 100% and a specificity of 85%. Coronary MRA is still undergoing rapid improvement, aimed to increase its accuracy for visualizing the distal coronary artery segments and to reduce the number of uninterpretable images. The key issue in coronary MRA to improve the image quality remains a trade-offs selection between various options to acquisition time, spatial resolution, CNR and correction of cardiac and respiratory motion. Parallel image encoding is one of the techniques to improve the acquisition speed. Multiple parallel imaging coil elements are used to simultaneously obtain the signal from region of interest. Each coil has a known specific sensitivity which needs to be mapped beforehand to calculate signal share by each coil. Parallel image encoding can be combined with common coronary MRA approaches like gradient echo and echo planar imaging. Potential disadvantages of parallel image encoding are the extended computation power, the requirement for pre-scanning (to create the sensitivity map), the signal-to-noise penalty that comes with this technique, and potential inaccuracies in reconstruction. The preliminary works demonstrated the feasibility of parallel imaging for coronary MRA and ability to cut down the acquisition time by half when using three-dimensional coronary MRA combined with respiratory navigator motion correction and parallel imaging as compared to a conventional approach. In summary, the main rationale for the application of parallel-image encoding techniques is the improved data acquisition speed, which in turn may allow achieve higher spatial resolution, lower temporal resolution, or larger three-dimensional volumes.

Spiral coronary MRA is another way to improve the image acquisition speed, in which the k-space is sampled more efficiently and faster. Spiral k-space sampling offers number of advantages [39;40]: 1) reduced acquisition speed by faster sampling, 2) enhanced contrast as sampling starts from the centre of the k-space, 3) acquisition are insensitive to flow artefacts. There are certain drawbacks with spiral MRS: 1) reduced SNR because of faster acquisition, 2) it is sensitive to main field inhomogeneity.

Steady State Free Precession (SSFP) in the sequence to improve the image contrast for coronary angiography [39;40]. It gives an excellent image contrast between blood and myocardium. SSFP is characterized by an alternating phase of excitation pulse combined with the application of time balanced gradients for all gradient directions. SSFP provides high signal intensity for tissues with a high T2/T1 ratio (blood) independent of TR and flow artefacts. SSFP is of special interest in cardiac functional analysis. SSFP has been compared with GRE, and improved endocardial border delineation was reported for the SSFP images which in turn facilitated automated edge detection during cardiac functional analysis. The potential use of SSFP for coronary MRA has recently been shown by Deshpande et al. in a study comparing conventional FLASH (fast low-angle shot) to three-dimensional true-FISP (Fast Imaging with Steady-state free Precession)[39]. The SNR and CNR were improved with 55% and 178% respectively for the SSFP acquisitions. McCarthy et al. used SSFP for the evaluation of coronary artery stenosis in 17 patients, with x-ray angiography as standard of reference. In this work, it was shown that hemodynamically significant stenoses could be detected with a sensitivity of 70% and a specificity of 88%.

Coronary MRA using a static magnetic field strength of 3 Tesla improves the signal-to-noise ratio, which in turn can be employed to increase the in-plane resolution, reduce the slice thickness, reduce the overall acquisition time, or to compensate for the signal-to-noise penalty that comes with several fast acquisition techniques such as echo planar imaging (EPI) or spiral imaging due to high sampling bandwidths. The increased field strength may also cause various side effects, especially when subjects move through the static field while entering the bore of the magnet leading to vertigo and nausea.

Cardiac motion correction is one major concern which captures much attention in cardiac MRA. Cardiac motion occurs in both systole and diastole, but is said to be minimal in mid-diastole (at diastasis). Cardiac motion correction is therefore usually achieved by timing the acquisition to the mid-diastolic phase of the cardiac cycle. There is considerable variation of motion patterns, motion ranges and motion velocities for coronary artery segments among individual patients. On average, the right coronary artery has greater movement and greater velocity as compared with the other coronary arteries, up to a factor of two for the proximal segments. But, inspite of all movements, the coronary arteries return to the same location from heartbeat to heartbeat during the rest period, which is an absolute requirement to perform a quality coronary MRA.

In addition to cardiac motion, heart is subjected to respiratory motions as well. Heart sits on the diaphragm, it translates during each respiratory cycle in a supero-inferior direction. These motion artefacts can be corrected and presently there are two approaches in clinical settings: 1) breath holding and 2) free-breathing navigator gating. During navigator gating approach, the position of the right hemi-diaphragm is deduced in real time from a navigator pencil beam acquisition. The image data that is acquired only while diaphragm position is within acceptable window are used for filling the k-space. The gating window is usually chosen as the end expiratory respiratory phase. Navigator implies that only a fraction of total imaging time is used for actual data acquisition. The lead to an overall imaging time prolonged by a factor of two using gating for motion correction. Patient compliance is very important in this aspect, an average navigator efficacy is 40-60% but it drops to 20%-30% when patient is in-compliant or very sick to maintain a regular breathing. The problem is sometime addressed with motion adapted gating (stringent acceptance window for low frequencies of k-space but wider window while acquiring higher frequencies).

Coronary MRA is practically used for all cardiac assessment protocols. Anomalous coronary arteries, coronary stenosis, bypass grafting and assessment of relative perfusion and vascular integrity are some of the commonest indications for cardiac MRA.

In conclusion, today's technical achievements for three-dimensional coronary MRA are able to provide excellent high-resolution images. However, MRA is still hampered by poor sensitivity and specificity for diagnosing coronary artery disease in distal segments even though it is the best non-invasive technique for evaluation of the proximal arteries. As coronary plaque imaging is still very challenging with MRA therefore CT Angiography benefits from high contrast of plaque compared to adjacent tissue even in the distal part of the coronary artery. However, with metal stents the major drawback in CT is, that the metal artifacts make image interpretation impossible.

7. Magnetic resonance angiography of the abdomen and pelvic arteries

Contrast enhancer MRA is now very well accepted as a reliable technique in assessment of abdominal vascular system (Figure 2 courtesy) [62]. In recent investigations, multiphase 3D CE-MRA has been shown advantageous in several respects [41;42]. The acquisition of multiple phases during contrast media transit guarantees the arterial contrast with no venous contamination [43;44]. In recent investigations with a more technical focus, multiphase 3D-Gd-MRA has been shown advantageous in several respects [45]. It is also shown that Time-resolved CE-MRA performed at 3 T with a 32-channel volume coil can be improved using the high-relaxivity agent, which increases quality and quantity of vessel enhancement (Figure 3 courtesy) [46].

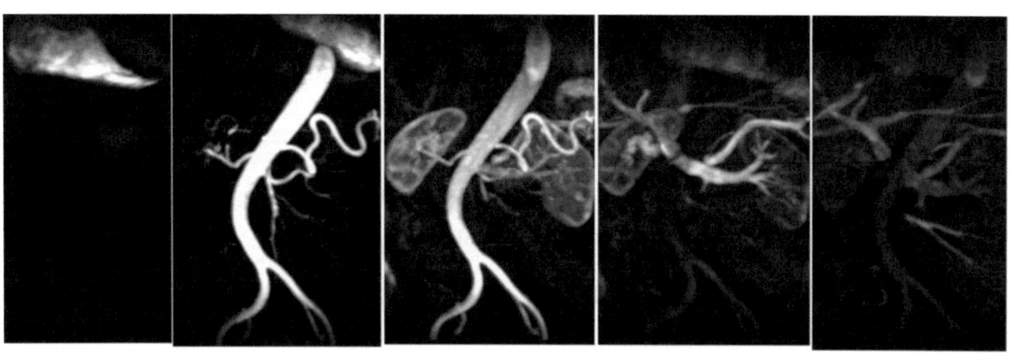

Fig. 2. Multiphasic MRA of abdominal aorta after injection of MR contrast Gd-BOPTA, showing arterial, parenchymal and venous phase with repect to time (sec).

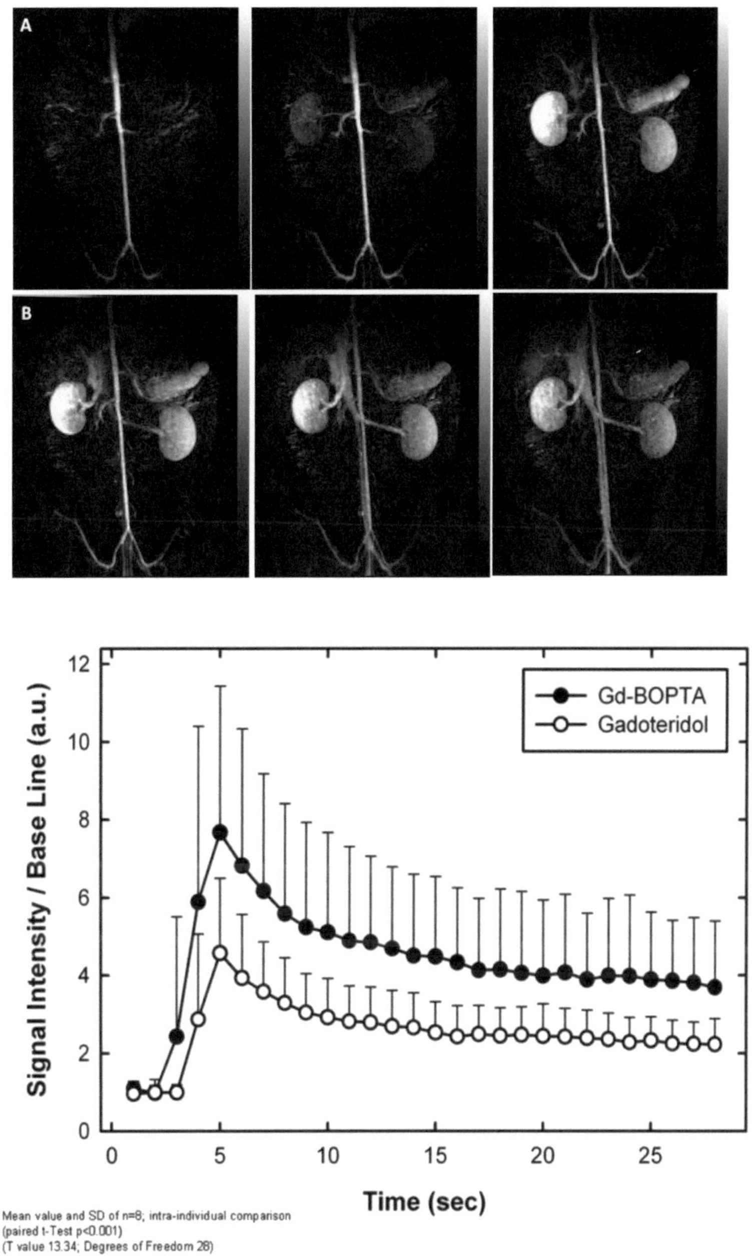

Fig. 3. Multiphasic time resolved CE-MRA allowed high spatial resolution imaging of the abdominal aorta. The first three phases present the early and late arterial phase while the lower row shows the early and late venous phase. The hepato-biliary pathway can be depicted nicely by Gd-BOPTA (a), while Gadoteridol is mainly excreted via the kidney (b). c) Relative signal time curve of both contrast media (SI [aorta] / SI [baseline]). Significantly ($p<0.001$; paired t-test) greater signal intensity enhancement was noted for Gd-BOPTA at all time-points after the peak signal enhancement is attained.

The acquisition of multiple phases during contrast media transit almost guarantees high arterial contrast with absent venous enhancement. In addition, the technique can show vessel segments with substantially delayed enhancement on successive scans. This is particularly important in cases of aortic dissection, aneurysm, or occlusion with variably delayed fill-in of the arteries downstream [47]. During a typical abdominal aorta imaging, in the early arterial phase, the distal and intrarenal arteries are visualized without substantial overlay from enhanced renal parenchyma [37]. In addition, vessels structures with delayed enhancement can be detected in later phases of the scan [48] [49]. It has been observed that the results from the renal arteries and common iliac arteries were somewhat better than those from the external iliac vessels and further distal segments [50]. This is most likely related to the three issues. First, the external iliac arteries curve fairly anteriorly and thus are often located in the margins of the 3D slab where the signal is typically inhomogeneous due to the poor slice profile of the fast 3D GRE sequences. Second, stenoses in this vessel's segments might be already located at the margin of the field-of-view where the magnetic field is not linear any more, resulting in image distortions [51;52]. Third, the spatial resolution of MRA sequence occasionally limits accurate evaluation of very small external iliac arteries [53]. In literature it has been reported that the acquisition of multiple phases is helpful for depicting vessel segments with substantially altered enhancement kinetics or delayed contrast fill-in [42;54]. Multiphase MRA is a robust technique with reproducible accuracy [31;43]. It can therefore be recommended for screening of atherosclerotic abdominal and pelvic arterial disease. Higher resolution MRA techniques may be preferred for staging of very small vessels, presurgical evaluation or fibromuscular disease.

8. Magnetic resonance angiography of vascular run-off

Contrast-Enhanced Magnetic Resonance Angiography is rapidly gaining acceptance as the method of choice for diagnostic imaging of the run-off vessels [55] [56] (Figure 4 courtesy [55]).

Compared with time-of-flight imaging, CE-MRA is significantly faster and far less prone to flow, saturation, and motion artefacts. Recent studies have shown CE-MRA with gadolinium contrast agents to be equivalent to conventional angiography for diagnostic imaging of the peripheral vasculature [57;58]. However, a problem inherent to CE-MRA of the run-off vessels is the large vascular territory to be imaged [56]. While technological improvements such as moving bed and dedicated lower extremity coils have contributed towards advances, satisfactory imaging of the run-off vessels is still highly dependent on the spatial resolution attainable. Unfortunately, spatial resolution in the peripheral arteries often is restricted by insufficient signal-to-noise (SNR) and contrast-to-noise (CNR) in the more distal parts of the field of view (FOV). In looking to overcome problems associated with insufficient SNR and CNR, various authors have advocated either single injections of high-dose contrast agents or cumulative dosing with injections at two or more stations along the vascular territory. Drawbacks of these approaches, however, include increased costs for contrast agents and, when multiple dosing protocols are used, problems associated with degraded image quality following the second injection due to residual gadolinium from the first injection and the high dose related Nephrogenic Systemic Fibrosis. An alternative approach to increasing SNR and CNR with standard doses of gadolinium without further

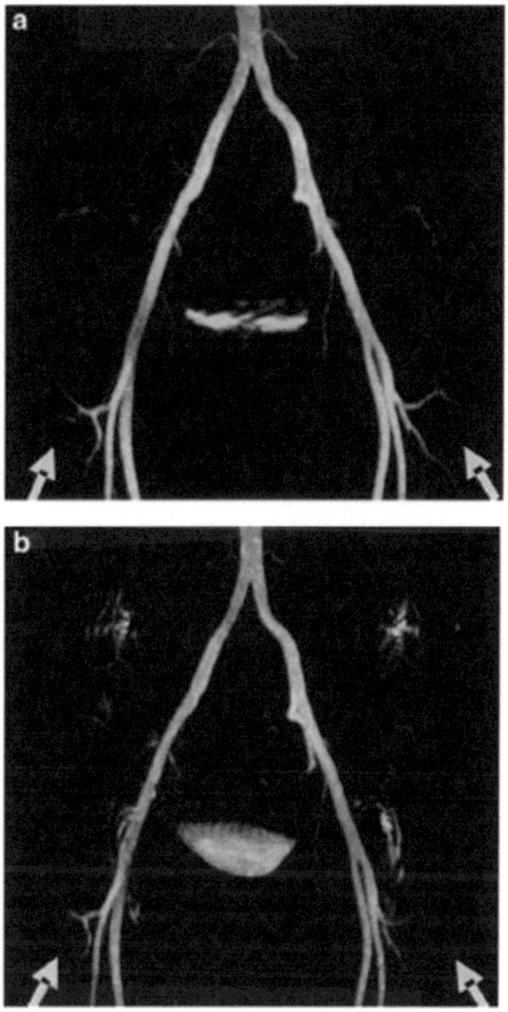

Fig. 4. Targeted maximum intensity projections (MIP) of the pelvic region in the same volunteer after identical dosing (0.1 mmol/kg bodyweight, flow rate of 0.8 mL/second, flush 25 mL saline) of the weakly protein interacting agent, Gd-BOPTA (a) in comparison to Gd-DTPA (b). The intra-individual comparison revealed better conspicuity of smaller vessels (arrows) as well as more homogenous vascular enhancement after Gd-BOPTA.

limiting spatial resolution would be to use contrast agents with preferential vascular contrasting properties. Gadobenate dimeglumine (Gd-BOPTA, MultiHance™; Bracco Imaging SpA, Milan, Italy) is a gadolinium based contrast agent that possesses increased T1 relaxivity in vivo compared to other available gadolinium agents (9.7 mM^{-1} $second^{-1}$ compared to between 4.3 and 5.0 mM^{-1} $second^{-1}$) due to a capacity for weak and transient interaction with serum albumin [59-61]. Preliminary investigations in healthy volunteers revealed that the vascular signal intensity of the abdominal aorta is higher and longer-lasting following administration of Gd-BOPTA than following administration of Gd-DTPA at the same dose and injection rate. More recently, studies in patient volunteers have demonstrated marked superiority of Gd-BOPTA over Gd-DTPA for time-resolved renal and pelvic CE-MRA [37]. Superiority for multiphasic MRA of the abdomen has also been noted for Gd-BOPTA compared to Gd-DTPA and the more highly concentrated gadolinium agent, Gd-BT-DO3A [56].

The trade-off between high spatial resolution and the need for sufficient SNR and CNR for successful diagnosis is particularly pronounced for CE-MRA of the run-off vessels. Currently, CE-MRA is most frequently performed using conventional gadolinium-based contrast agents such as Gd-DTPA whose T1 relaxivities in protein-containing aqueous solution fall in the range between 4.3 and 5.0 mM^{-1} $second^{-1}$. These agents possess no capacity for protein interaction and it is frequently necessary to use comparatively high doses or cumulative dosing regimens to obtain sufficient diagnostic quality along the length of the peripheral vasculature. Since the diagnostic quality of CE-MRA is dependent upon the intensity of vascular contrast and thus the extent to which the T1 relaxation time in blood is reduced during image acquisition, contrast agents with higher T1 relaxivity in blood may be expected to provide greater vascular signal intensity enhancement and hence greater diagnostic efficacy. Gd-BOPTA is a gadolinium-based MR contrast agent whose plasma kinetics are indistinguishable from those of Gd-DTPA and other non-specific gadolinium-based contrast agents in demonstrating complete elimination within 3 days of administration. The results of these studies confirm the superiority of Gd-BOPTA over Gd-DTPA for CE-MRA; significantly higher CNR and SNR were noted for Gd- BOPTA for almost all segments from the distal 2 cm of the abdominal aorta to the posterior and anterior tibial arteries [35;62]. The only segment for which statistical superiority have not been demonstrated was the right iliac artery. That superiority was not demonstrated for this vessel can be attributed to the fact that an unusually wide range of values were noted for this segment compared to the other eight segments. It is possible that this was due to this region lying at the edge of the field of view and the coil as mentioned earlier. In terms of the diagnostic quality of images acquired, the results of the studies again indicate superiority for Gd-BOPTA [63]; the overall diagnostic quality score out of a maximum possible score of 18 was 17.4 ± 1.5 for Gd-BOPTA and 13.8 ± 2.4 for Gd-DTPA [64] [63]. Significantly, there were no vascular segments in which diagnostic quality was determined to be poor following Gd-BOPTA administration [63]. On the other hand sometimes diagnostic quality was determined to be poor for the left and right tibio-fibular trunks of four of the fourteen subjects (28.6%) following Gd-DTPA administration in a study. Venous overlay is a potential problem for long time of acquisition. The availability of sequences with shorter TR and TE time which permit more rapid acquisitions may go some way towards overcoming potential problems of venous overlay when using Gd-BOPTA for peripheral MRA [63]. The greatest benefits of Gd-BOPTA are to be found in the most distal, smaller vessels of the lower leg [63]. In terms of its potential usefulness in routine clinical practice, one possibility is that a lower overall dose could be employed to achieve similar increases in SNR and CNR to those increases currently achieved with Gd-DTPA at the same dose. Higher doses of Gd-DTPA and other conventional agents, and a variety of dosing regimens, are currently used to evaluate patients with peripheral vascular disease. Future work might usefully be aimed at evaluating whether better diagnostic performance is achievable with equivalent high doses of Gd-BOPTA or whether lower overall doses can be employed satisfactorily [65]. Similarly, it would be of interest to determine more precisely the influence of injection rate on Gd-BOPTA-enhanced MRA of the peripheral arteries.

9. References

[1] Sadowski EA, Bennett LK, Chan MR, et al. Nephrogenic systemic fibrosis: risk factors and incidence estimation. Radiology 2007; 243:148-157

[2] Broome DR, Girguis MS, Baron PW, Cottrell AC, Kjellin I, Kirk GA. Gadodiamide-associated nephrogenic systemic fibrosis: why radiologists should be concerned. AJR Am J Roentgenol 2007; 188:586-592

[3] Klessen C, Hein PA, Huppertz A, et al. First-pass whole-body magnetic resonance angiography (MRA) using the blood-pool contrast medium gadofosveset trisodium: comparison to gadopentetate dimeglumine. Invest Radiol 2007; 42:659-664

[4] Goyen M. Gadofosveset-enhanced magnetic resonance angiography. Vasc Health Risk Manag 2008; 4:1-9

[5] Heverhagen JT, Bourekas E, Sammet S, Knopp MV, Schmalbrock P. Time-of-flight magnetic resonance angiography at 7 Tesla. Invest Radiol 2008; 43:568-573

[6] de HC, Cabrini M, Akhnana L, Ratti D, Calabi L, Gozzini L. Gadobenate dimeglumine 0.5 M solution for injection (MultiHance) pharmaceutical formulation and physicochemical properties of a new magnetic resonance imaging contrast medium. J Comput Assist Tomogr 1999; 23 Suppl 1:S161-S168

[7] Pintaske J, Martirosian P, Graf H, et al. Relaxivity of Gadopentetate Dimeglumine (Magnevist), Gadobutrol (Gadovist), and Gadobenate Dimeglumine (MultiHance) in human blood plasma at 0.2, 1.5, and 3 Tesla. Invest Radiol 2006; 41:213-221

[8] Giesel FL, Mehndiratta A, Essig M. High-relaxivity contrast-enhanced magnetic resonance neuroimaging: a review. Eur Radiol 2010; 20:2461-2474

[9] Rohrer M, Bauer H, Mintorovitch J, Requardt M, Weinmann HJ. Comparison of magnetic properties of MRI contrast media solutions at different magnetic field strengths. Invest Radiol 2005; 40:715-724

[10] Korosec FR, Frayne R, Grist TM, Mistretta CA. Time-resolved contrast-enhanced 3D MR angiography. Magn Reson Med 1996; 36:345-351

[11] Fink C, Goyen M, Lotz J. Magnetic resonance angiography with blood-pool contrast agents: future applications. Eur Radiol 2007; 17 Suppl 2:B38-B44

[12] Essig M, Weber MA, von Tengg-Kobligk H, Knopp MV, Yuh WT, Giesel FL. Contrast-enhanced magnetic resonance imaging of central nervous system tumors: agents, mechanisms, and applications. Top Magn Reson Imaging 2006; 17:89-106

[13] Pomper MG, Port JD. New techniques in MR imaging of brain tumors. Magn Reson Imaging Clin N Am 2000; 8:691-713

[14] Cotton F, Hermier M. The advantage of high relaxivity contrast agents in brain perfusion. Eur Radiol 2006; 16 Suppl 7:M16-M26

[15] Knopp MV, Runge VM, Essig M, et al. Primary and secondary brain tumors at MR imaging: bicentric intraindividual crossover comparison of gadobenate dimeglumine and gadopentetate dimeglumine. Radiology 2004; 230:55-64

[16] Kuhn MJ, Picozzi P, Maldjian JA, et al. Evaluation of intraaxial enhancing brain tumors on magnetic resonance imaging: intraindividual crossover comparison of gadobenate dimeglumine and gadopentetate dimeglumine for visualization and assessment, and implications for surgical intervention. J Neurosurg 2007; 106:557-566

[17] Lev MH, Rosen BR. Clinical applications of intracranial perfusion MR imaging. Neuroimaging Clin N Am 1999; 9:309-331

[18] Caravan P. Protein-targeted gadolinium-based magnetic resonance imaging (MRI) contrast agents: design and mechanism of action. Acc Chem Res 2009; 42:851-862

[19] Caravan P, Farrar CT, Frullano L, Uppal R. Influence of molecular parameters and increasing magnetic field strength on relaxivity of gadolinium- and manganese-based T1 contrast agents. Contrast Media Mol Imaging 2009; 4:89-100

[20] Bueltmann E, Erb G, Kirchin MA, Klose U, Naegele T. Intra-individual crossover comparison of gadobenate dimeglumine and gadopentetate dimeglumine for contrast-enhanced magnetic resonance angiography of the supraaortic vessels at 3 Tesla. Invest Radiol 2008; 43:695-702

[21] Pediconi F, Fraioli F, Catalano C, et al. Gadobenate dimeglumine (Gd-DTPA) vs gadopentetate dimeglumine (Gd-BOPTA) for contrast-enhanced magnetic resonance angiography (MRA): improvement in intravascular signal intensity and contrast to noise ratio. Radiol Med 2003; 106:87-93

[22] Jourdan C, Heverhagen JT, Knopp MV. Dose comparison of single- vs. double-dose in contrast-enhanced magnetic resonance angiography of the carotid arteries: Intraindividual cross-over blinded trial using Gd-DTPA. J Magn Reson Imaging 2007; 25:557-563

[23] Giesel FL, Mehndiratta A, Risse F, et al. Intraindividual comparison between gadopentetate dimeglumine and gadobutrol for magnetic resonance perfusion in normal brain and intracranial tumors at 3 Tesla. Acta Radiol 2009; 50:521-530

[24] Essig M, Nikolaou K, Meaney JF. Magnetic resonance angiography of the head and neck vessels. Eur Radiol 2007; 17 Suppl 2:B30-B37

[25] Boxerman JL, Hamberg LM, Rosen BR, Weisskoff RM. MR contrast due to intravascular magnetic susceptibility perturbations. Magn Reson Med 1995; 34:555-566

[26] Boxerman JL, Rosen BR, Weisskoff RM. Signal-to-noise analysis of cerebral blood volume maps from dynamic NMR imaging studies. J Magn Reson Imaging 1997; 7:528-537

[27] Tombach B, Benner T, Reimer P, et al. Do highly concentrated gadolinium chelates improve MR brain perfusion imaging? Intraindividually controlled randomized crossover concentration comparison study of 0.5 versus 1.0 mol/L gadobutrol. Radiology 2003; 226:880-888

[28] Tombach B, Heindel W. Value of 1.0- M gadolinium chelates: review of preclinical and clinical data on gadobutrol. Eur Radiol 2002; 12:1550-1556

[29] Tombach B, Bohndorf K, Brodtrager W, et al. Comparison of 1.0 M gadobutrol and 0.5 M gadopentate dimeglumine-enhanced MRI in 471 patients with known or suspected renal lesions: results of a multicenter, single-blind, interindividual, randomized clinical phase III trial. Eur Radiol 2008; 18:2610-2619

[30] Prince MR, Narasimham DL, Stanley JC, et al. Breath-hold gadolinium-enhanced MR angiography of the abdominal aorta and its major branches. Radiology 1995; 197:785-792

[31] Schoenberg SO, Bock M, Floemer F, et al. High-resolution pulmonary arterio- and venography using multiple-bolus multiphase 3D-Gd-mRA. J Magn Reson Imaging 1999; 10:339-346

[32] Meaney JF, Weg JG, Chenevert TL, Stafford-Johnson D, Hamilton BH, Prince MR. Diagnosis of pulmonary embolism with magnetic resonance angiography. N Engl J Med 1997; 336:1422-1427

[33] Sloop RD, Lium JH. Systemic arterial embolism arising from pulmonary thrombophlebitis. Am Surg 1971; 37:503-505

[34] Schoenberg SO, Knopp MV, Grau A, et al. [Ultrafast MRI phlebography of the lungs]. Radiologe 1998; 38:597-605
[35] von Tengg-Kobligk H, Floemer F, Knopp MV. [Multiphasic MR angiography as an intra-individual comparison between the contrast agents Gd-DTPA, Gd-BOPTA, and Gd-BT-DO3A]. Radiologe 2003; 43:171-178
[36] Lee CH, Goo JM, Bae KT, et al. CTA contrast enhancement of the aorta and pulmonary artery: the effect of saline chase injected at two different rates in a canine experimental model. Invest Radiol 2007; 42:486-490
[37] Dong Q, Schoenberg SO, Carlos RC, et al. Diagnosis of renal vascular disease with MR angiography. Radiographics 1999; 19:1535-1554
[38] Kim WY, Danias PG, Stuber M, et al. Coronary magnetic resonance angiography for the detection of coronary stenoses. N Engl J Med 2001; 345:1863-1869
[39] Deshpande VS, Shea SM, Laub G, Simonetti OP, Finn JP, Li D. 3D magnetization-prepared true-FISP: a new technique for imaging coronary arteries. Magn Reson Med 2001; 46:494-502
[40] Dirksen MS, Lamb HJ, Doornbos J, Bax JJ, Jukema JW, de RA. Coronary magnetic resonance angiography: technical developments and clinical applications. J Cardiovasc Magn Reson 2003; 5:365-386
[41] Glockner JF. Three-dimensional gadolinium-enhanced MR angiography: applications for abdominal imaging. Radiographics 2001; 21:357-370
[42] Schoenberg SO, Bock M, Knopp MV, et al. Renal arteries: optimization of three-dimensional gadolinium-enhanced MR angiography with bolus-timing-independent fast multiphase acquisition in a single breath hold. Radiology 1999; 211:667-679
[43] Schoenberg SO, Essig M, Hallscheidt P, et al. Multiphase magnetic resonance angiography of the abdominal and pelvic arteries: results of a bicenter multireader analysis. Invest Radiol 2002; 37:20-28
[44] Shetty AN, Bis KG, Vrachliotis TG, Kirsch M, Shirkhoda A, Ellwood R. Contrast-enhanced 3D MRA with centric ordering in k space: a preliminary clinical experience in imaging the abdominal aorta and renal and peripheral arterial vasculature. J Magn Reson Imaging 1998; 8:603-615
[45] Yamashita Y, Mitsuzaki K, Ogata I, Takahashi M, Hiai Y. Three-dimensional high-resolution dynamic contrast-enhanced MR angiography of the pelvis and lower extremities with use of a phased array coil and subtraction: diagnostic accuracy. J Magn Reson Imaging 1998; 8:1066-1072
[46] Giesel FL, Runge V, Kirchin M, et al. Three-dimensional multiphase time-resolved low-dose contrast-enhanced magnetic resonance angiography using TWIST on a 32-channel coil at 3 T: a quantitative and qualitative comparison of a conventional gadolinium chelate with a high-relaxivity agent. J Comput Assist Tomogr 2010; 34:678-683
[47] Schoenberg SO, Wunsch C, Knopp MV, et al. Abdominal aortic aneurysm. Detection of multilevel vascular pathology by time-resolved multiphase 3D gadolinium MR angiography: initial report. Invest Radiol 1999; 34:648-659
[48] Sadick M, Diehl SJ, Lehmann KJ, Gaa J, Mockel R, Georgi M. Evaluation of breath-hold contrast-enhanced 3D magnetic resonance angiography technique for imaging visceral abdominal arteries and veins. Invest Radiol 2000; 35:111-117
[49] Schoenberg SO, Knopp MV, Prince MR, Londy F, Knopp MA. Arterial-phase three-dimensional gadolinium magnetic resonance angiography of the renal arteries.

Strategies for timing and contrast media injection: original investigation. Invest Radiol 1998; 33:506-514
[50] Heverhagen JT, Wright CL, Schmalbrock P, Knopp MV. Dose comparison of single versus double dose in contrast-enhanced magnetic resonance angiography of the renal arteries: intra-individual cross-over blinded trial using Gd-DTPA. Eur Radiol 2009; 19:67-72
[51] Volk M, Strotzer M, Lenhart M, et al. Time-resolved contrast-enhanced MR angiography of renal artery stenosis: diagnostic accuracy and interobserver variability. AJR Am J Roentgenol 2000; 174:1583-1588
[52] Gilfeather M, Yoon HC, Siegelman ES, et al. Renal artery stenosis: evaluation with conventional angiography versus gadolinium-enhanced MR angiography. Radiology 1999; 210:367-372
[53] Winterer JT, Laubenberger J, Scheffler K, et al. Contrast-enhanced subtraction MR angiography in occlusive disease of the pelvic and lower limb arteries: results of a prospective intraindividual comparative study with digital subtraction angiography in 76 patients. J Comput Assist Tomogr 1999; 23:583-589
[54] Boos M, Lentschig M, Scheffler K, Bongartz GM, Steinbrich W. Contrast-enhanced magnetic resonance angiography of peripheral vessels. Different contrast agent applications and sequence strategies: a review. Invest Radiol 1998; 33:538-546
[55] Knopp MV, Giesel FL, von Tengg-Kobligk H, et al. Contrast-enhanced MR angiography of the run-off vasculature: intraindividual comparison of gadobenate dimeglumine with gadopentetate dimeglumine. J Magn Reson Imaging 2003; 17:694-702
[56] Ho KY, Leiner T, van Engelshoven JM. MR angiography of run-off vessels. Eur Radiol 1999; 9:1285-1289
[57] Quinn SF, Sheley RC, Semonsen KG, Leonardo VJ, Kojima K, Szumowski J. Aortic and lower-extremity arterial disease: evaluation with MR angiography versus conventional angiography. Radiology 1998; 206:693-701
[58] Vosshenrich R, Kopka L, Castillo E, Bottcher U, Graessner J, Grabbe E. Electrocardiograph-triggered two-dimensional time-of-flight versus optimized contrast-enhanced three-dimensional MR angiography of the peripheral arteries. Magn Reson Imaging 1998; 16:887-892
[59] Ruehm SG, Hany TF, Pfammatter T, Schneider E, Ladd M, Debatin JF. Pelvic and lower extremity arterial imaging: diagnostic performance of three-dimensional contrast-enhanced MR angiography. AJR Am J Roentgenol 2000; 174:1127-1135
[60] Ruehm SG, Nanz D, Baumann A, Schmid M, Debatin JF. 3D contrast-enhanced MR angiography of the run-off vessels: value of image subtraction. J Magn Reson Imaging 2001; 13:402-411
[61] Catalano C, Pediconi F, Nardis P, et al. MR angiography with MultiHance for imaging the supra-aortic vessels. Eur Radiol 2004; 14 Suppl 7:O45-O51
[62] Knopp MV, Schoenberg SO, Rehm C, et al. Assessment of gadobenate dimeglumine for magnetic resonance angiography: phase I studies. Invest Radiol 2002; 37:706-715
[63] Herborn CU, Lauenstein TC, Ruehm SG, Bosk S, Debatin JF, Goyen M. Intraindividual comparison of gadopentetate dimeglumine, gadobenate dimeglumine, and gadobutrol for pelvic 3D magnetic resonance angiography. Invest Radiol 2003; 38:27-33
[64] Earls JP, Patel NH, Smith PA, DeSena S, Meissner MH. Gadolinium-enhanced three-dimensional MR angiography of the aorta and peripheral arteries: evaluation of a multistation examination using two gadopentetate dimeglumine infusions. AJR Am J Roentgenol 1998; 171:599-604
[65] Knopp MV, von Tengg-Kobligk H, Floemer F, Schoenberg SO. Contrast agents for MRA: future directions. J Magn Reson Imaging 1999; 10:314-316

Part 2

Intracranial MRA Advances and Future Prospectives

3

Intracranial Plaque Imaging Using High-Resolution Magnetic Resonance Imaging: A Pictorial Review

Kuniyasu Niizuma, Hiroaki Shimizu and Teiji Tominaga
Department of Neurosurgery, Tohoku University Graduate School of Medicine, Sendai, Japan

1. Introduction

Intracranial atherosclerotic disease is defined as the development, progression, and complication of atherosclerotic lesions on intracranial large arteries. It has been considered to be the most common cause of ischemic stroke worldwide (Gorelick et al., 2008; Kim et al, 2006; Won et al., 1998).

Intracranial atherosclerotic disease is normally detected by hemodynamically relevant intracranial stenosis using luminography-based methods. However, from the extracranial study, it is well known that lumen diameter can be maintained due to remodeling of the arteries in spite of wall thickening (Glagov et al., 1987), suggesting conventional luminography-based methods might underestimate atherosclerotic disease. Arenillas (Arenillas, 2001) summarized limitations of conventional approach. First, it only detects advanced stage of intracranial atherosclerotic disease with luminal narrowing. Second, it cannot provide the histopathologic information of the intracranial atherosclerotic plaque. Third, it is unable to differentiate atherostenosis from stenosis caused by other entities.

Intracranial small infarctions result from atherosclerosis of the parent arteries, which may occlude the orifice of the perforating artery as branch atheromatous disease. Small infarctions also result from lipohyalinosis or microatheromatous, or embolic occlusion of a perforating artery (Adams et al., 1993; Cho et al., 2007; Donnan et al., 1991; Fisher, 1965, 1982). Since branch atheromatous disease is more aggressive than typical lacunar infarctions, intensive antiplatelette or anti-thrombic therapy may be needed for the treatment of branch atheromatous disease. However, the diagnosis of these small infarctions is still difficult because conventional techniques are limited to detect the plaque.

Studies regarding intracranial plaque image have achieved to reveal the mechanism of small infarctions or to diagnose early stage of intracranial atherosclerotic disease. In this report, we address such new magnetic resonance imaging techniques to detect intracranial plaques.

2. Intracranial plaque image

Recently, high-resolution magnetic resonance imaging has been reported to visualize intracranial atherosclerotic plaques (Klein et al., 2005, 2006; Niizuma et al., 2008). It can detect not only stenotic but nonstenotic intracranial atheromatous plaques or vessel wall thickning. It might provide the information regarding well-known determinants of plaque instability such as richer content in lipid, intraplaque hemorrhage and inflammatory cell infiltration (Chen et al., 2008)

For high-resolution magnetic resonance imaging, pulse sequences were varied. T1-weighted, T2-weighted, moderate T2-weighted, proton density-weighted, and/or postcontrast T1-weighted images by gadolinium-diethylenetriaminepenta-acetic acid with/without miuticontrast black blood sequences were used.

2.1 Basillar artery plaque imaging (Fig. 1)

The infarction mechanism of basilar perforating artery territory can be divided into branch atheromatous disease, cardiogenic embolism, and small vessel disease. Especially, basilar branch atheromatous disease is the most frequent cause of basilar perforating artery territory infarctions (Bassetti et al., 1996; Kumral et al., 2002). Basilar artery atheomatous plaque can block at the orifice of the branch, or can extend into the perforating branch, which results in parapontine or deep pontine infarctions (Fisher & Caplan, 1971; Fisher, 1977).

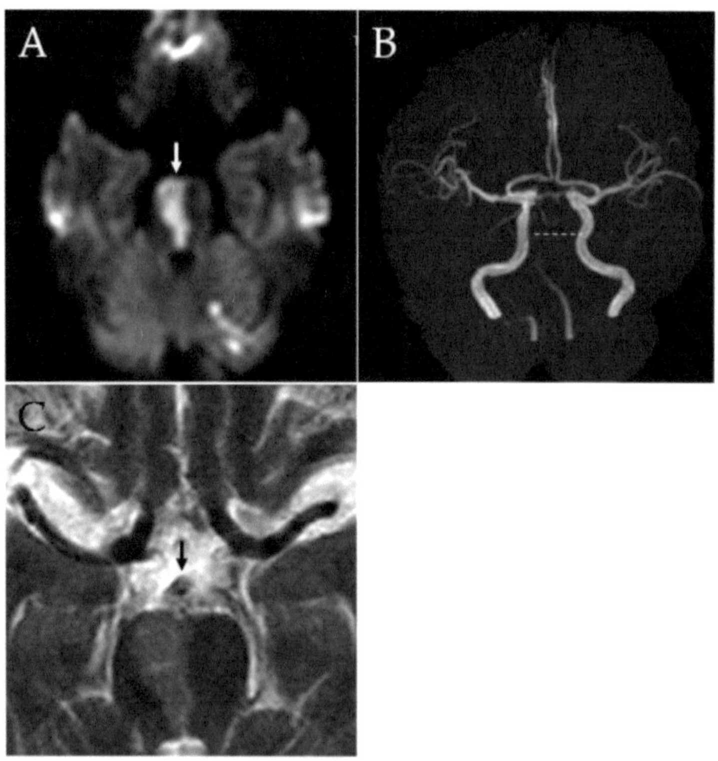

Fig. 1. Basilar artery plaque image using 1.5 tesla magnetic resonance imaging scanner. A: Axial diffusion-weighted image demonstrating a right paramedian pontine high-intensity lesion (arrow). B: Magnetic resonance angiography showing severe stenosis of the basilar artery. C: T2-weighted image at the level of the dotted line on B (TR/TE 3500/100, matrix size 254 × 320), presenting plaque on the vessel wall (arrow).

To detect basilar artery plaques of the basilar artery, Klein et al used high-resolution magnetic resonance imaging with a 1.5-tesla system (Klein et al., 2005, 2010). Twenty-four consecutive patients with the paramedian pontine infarctions underwent high-resolution magnetic resonance imaging, which revealed basilar atherosclerotic plaques in up to 70% patients. Plaque was identified in all patients with severe or moderate stenosis as well as in some patients with normal findings on magnetic resonance angiography (Klein et al., 2005).

Basilar artery plaque could also be a prevalent mechanism not only in the paramedianpontine infarctions but also lacunar or small deep pontine infarctions (Klein et al., 2010). High-resolution magnetic resonance imaging was performed on 43 consecutive patients of medial pontine infarct, including lacunar or small pontine infarction. Basilar artery plaque was detected in 73% of lacunar or small deep pontine infarction cases. This pattern was similar to the cases or paramedian pontine infarctions.

2.2 Middle cerebral artery plaque imaging (Fig. 2-4)

The infarct mechanism in the middle cerebral perforating arterial territory can be divided into four subtypes regardless of lesion size (Cho et al., 2007): (1) middle cerebral artery disease, if there is a corresponding ipsilateral atherosclerotic middle cerebral artery lesion without cardiogenic embolism or atherosclerotic lesion proximal to the middle cerebral artery lesion; (2) internal carotid artery disease, if there is significant ipsilateral internal carotid artery stenosis (> 50%) without evidence of middle cerebral artery disease or cardiogenic embolism; (3) cardiogenic embolism, if there is emboligenic heart disease based on stroke classification criteria developed by the investigators of the Trial of Org 10172 in Acute Stroke Treatment (Adams et al., 1993) in the absence of atherosclerotic diseases in cerebral vessels; and (4) small vessel disease, if there is no cardiogenic embolism, middle cerebral artery disease, or internal carotid artery disease. People with symptomatic middle cerebral artery disease have overall stroke risk of 12.5% per year (Kern et al., 2005). Since the outcome of middle cerebral artery disease was poor, diagnosis of middle cerebral artery disease is clinically important.

Middle cerebral artery plaque imaging was first reported by on 6 patients of severe middle cerebral artery stenosis using 1.5-tesla magnetic resonance imaging system (Klein et al., 2006). Plaque was clearly detected on the middle cerebral artery wall in all cases. Quantitative measurements presented that lumen area was significantly larger in normal middle cerebral artery segments compared with atherosclerotic ones.

Then several authors reported high-resolution magnetic resonance imaging with a 3-tesla system, by which they detected plaques on the middle cerebral artery and/or wall thickening (Li et al., 2009; Niizuma et al., 2008; Ryu et al., 2009; Swartz et al., 2009; Turan et al., 2011; Xu et al., 2010). Niizuma et al (Niizuma et al., 2008) demonstrated moderate T2-weighted high-resolution magnetic resonance imaging showed plaques on the middle cerebral artery in cases of corona radiate infarction, which indicated the etiology of the infarction (Fig. 2-4). Swartz et al (Swartz et al., 2009) presented that high-resolution magnetic resonance imaging may distinguish the enhancement patterns of different pathologies such as atherosclerosis, inflammation, and other pathologies of the intracranial vessel wall. Ryu et al (Ryu et al., 2009) found multicontrast-weighted black blood imaging have the potential to characterize atherosclerotic plaques. Li et al (Li et al., 2009) and Xu et al (Xu et al., 2010) demonstrated that T2-weighted high-resolution magnetic resonance

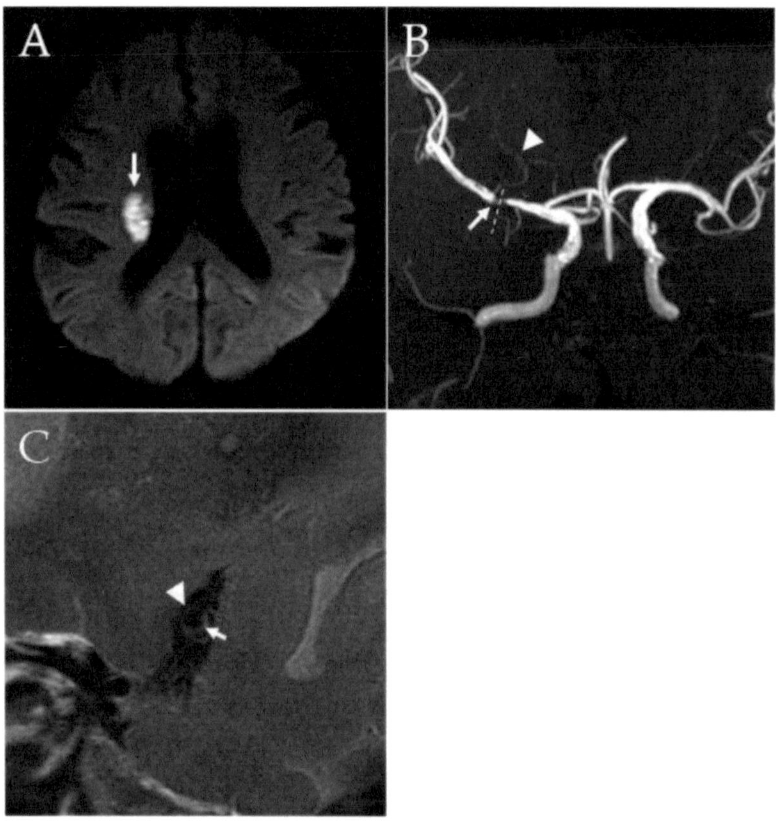

Fig. 2. Middle cerebral artery plaque which is also detected by magnetic resonance angiography (modified from Niizuma et al., 2008). A: Axial diffusion-weighted image demonstrating a high-intensity lesion, 20 mm in diameter, in the right corona radiata (arrow). B: Magnetic resonance angiography processed by partial maximum intensity projection indicating the relationship between the stenotic area (arrow) and lateral striate arteries (arrowhead). C: High-resolution magnetic resonance image perpendicular to the right MCA, at the level of the dotted line on B (TR/TE 2800/50.8, FOV 12 cm × 12 cm, matrix size 512 × 256, slice thickness 2 mm, interslice gap 0.3 mm, NEX 5), presenting the lumen of the right middle cerebral artery (arrow) and plaque on the vessel wall (arrowhead).

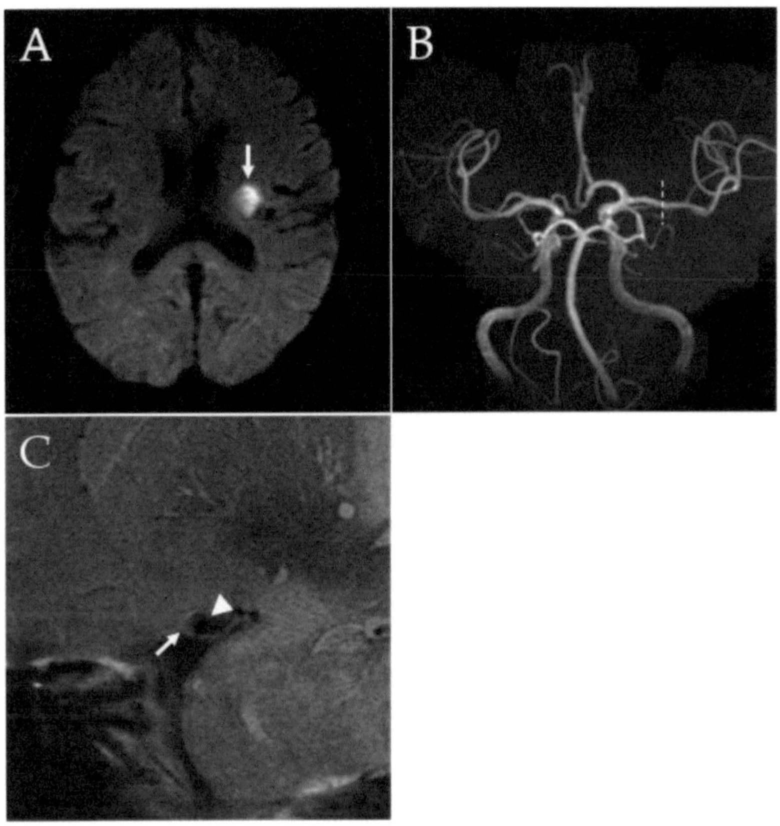

Fig. 3. Middle cerebral artery plaque which cannot be detected by magnetic resonance angiography (modified from Niizuma et al., 2008). A: Axial Diffusion-weighted image demonstrating a high-intensity lesion, 12 mm in diameter, in the left corona radiata (arrow). B: Magnetic resonance angiography showing no evidence of atherosclerosis. C: High-resolution magnetic resonance image perpendicular to the left MCA, at the level of the dotted line in B (TR/TE 2800/50.8, FOV 12 cm × 12 cm, matrix size 512 × 256, slice thickness 2 mm, interslice gap 0.3 mm, NEX 5), presenting the lumen of the left middle cerebral artery (arrow) and plaque on the vessel wall (arrowhead), despite the apparently normal magnetic resonance angiography.

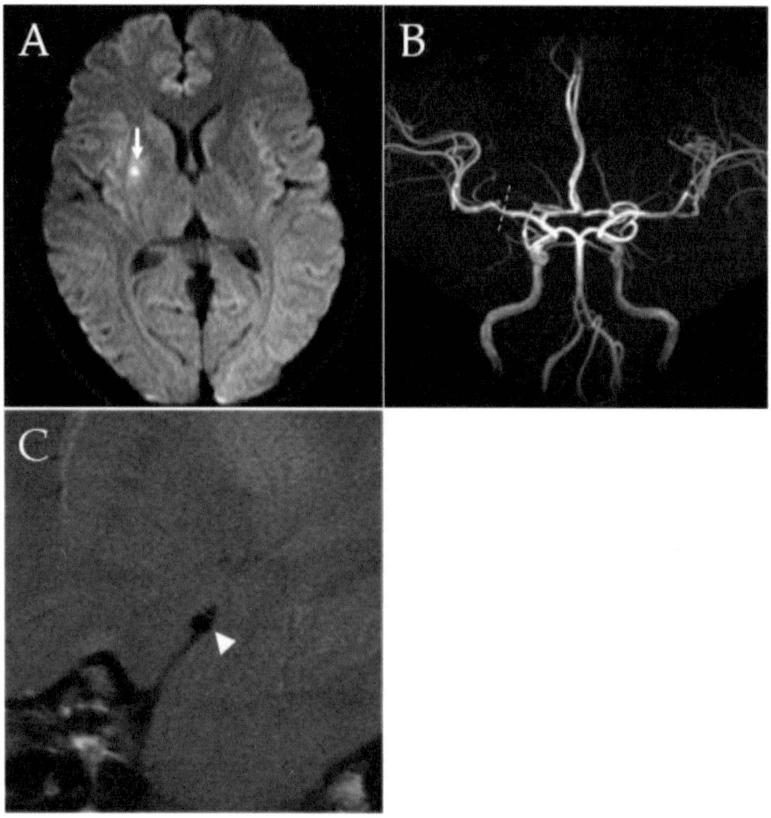

Fig. 4. No detection of middlee cerebral artery plaque on the right lacunar infarction (modified from Niizuma et al., 2008). Axial Diffusion-weighted image demonstrating a high-intensity lesion in the right putamen (arrow) and corona radiate. B: Magnetic resonance angiography showing no evidence of atherosclerosis. C: High-resolution magnetic resonance image perpendicular to the right middle cerebral artery, at the level of the dotted line in B (TR/TE 2800/50.8, FOV 12 cm × 12 cm, matrix size 512 × 256, slice thickness 2 mm, interslice gap 0.3 mm, NEX 5), presenting the lumen of the middle cerebral artery (arrowhead), though there were no plaques on the vessel wall.

imaging differentiated wall thickening, arterial remodeling, and atherosclerotic plaque in symptomatic and asymptomatic patients with intracranial middle cerebral artery stenosis.

2.3 High-field magnetic resonance imaging

Although 3.0-tesla magnetic resonance imaging clearly demonstrated plaques and abnormal intracranial vessel walls, it seemed difficult to show the healthy vessel wall (Li et al., 2009; Niizuma et al., 2008; Ryu et al., 2009; Swartz et al., 2009; Turan et al., 2011; Xu et al., 2010). Van der Kolk et al (Van der Kolk et al., 2011) aimed to depict the vessel wall of intracranial arteries, also in the absence of disease. They used a volumetric turbo spin-echo sequence with inversion recovery and magnetization preparation using 7.0-tesla system. They achieved high image resolution and sensitivity, thus walls of major arteries of the circle of Willis were identified in all cases. 7.0-tesla high-resolution magnetic resonance imaging depicted that 66% of the patients had more than one lesions in major intracranial arteries, whereas only 27%of the lesions caused stenosis on magnetic resonance angiography. They concluded that 7.0-tesla high-resolution magnetic resonance imaging has possibility to study the role of intracranial arterial wall pathology in more detail.

2.4 Plaque instability

Richer content in lipid, intraplaque hemorrhage and inflammatory cell infiltration are well-known determinants of plaque instability (Chen et al., 2008). Now, magnetic resonance imaging has the ability to differentiate such plaque components in addition to determining the degree of luminal narrowing of the carotid plaques (Fayad & Fuster, 2000). The use of gadolinium-diethylenetriaminepenta-acetic acid may enhance detection of wall lesions and determination of plaque instability. In the caroted artery, plaque enhancement may indicate neovascularized fibrous tissue that correlates with unstable plaque (Yuan et al., 2002a). Multisequence magnetic resonance imaging can identify different carotid plaque components with high sensitivity, specificity, and accuracy not only ex vivo but also in vivo (Shinnar et al., 1999; Yuan et al., 2001). High-resolution magnetic resonance imaging of the carotid plaque can distinguish advanced lesions from early and intermediate atherosclerotic plaque (Cai et al., 2002).

As intracranial plaque instability, Meyers et al (Meyers et al., 2009) reported that intraplaque hemorrhage was detected by intravascular ultrasound in symptomatic intracranial atherosclerotic disease, indicating that intracranial atherosclerotic plaques can become symptomatic after complication by intraplaque hemorrhage similer to coronary artery plaques. Moreover, Turan et al (Turan et al., 2011) observed intraplaque high signal intensity lesion in the symptomatic middle cerebral artery stenosis using high-resolution T1-weighted image. Its characteristics were similer to intraplaque hemorrhage on the caroted arteries. These findings suggest that high-resolution magnetic resonance imaging allows characterization of intraplaque hemorrhage in vivo.

The diagnostic value of different enhanced patterns of intracranial plaques by gadolinium-diethylenetriaminepenta-acetic acid is not determined, although plaque enhancement is commonly considered to be a marker of symptomatic or unstable plaque. Swartz et al (Swartz et al., 2009) described that enhanced patterns of plaques might differentiate pathologies such as atherosclerosis, inflammation, and other pathologies of the intracranial vessel wall (Swartz et al., 2009). However, Klein et al (Klein et al., 2006) described a case of asymptomatic middle cerebral artery stenosisi with strongly enhanced plaque by gadolinium-diethylenetriaminepenta-acetic acid, indicating plaque enhancement does not always indicate symptomatic plaque. Further studies are needed to determine this issue.

2.5 Limitations

For clinical use of high-resolution magnetic resonance imaging to detect intracranial plaques, following issues must be considered. First, whether the plaque is a true plaque must be more confirmed. Other modalities such as ultrasound, pathology, or interaoperative observation should be compared with findings of high-resolution magnetic resonance image. Although previous studies of carotid artery plaques demonstrated a significant correlation between pathological findings and plaque characteristics detected by high-resolution magnetic resonance imaging (Honda et al., 2006; Toussaint et al., 1996; Yuan et al., 2002b), histological analyses are required to evaluate this technique in detail.

Second, high-resolution magnetic resonance imaging cannot demonstrate a direct causative relationship between plaque and infarctions, even if plaques are located at the level of the perforating arteries. Because of the small size of intracranial arteries, spatial resolution needs to be more optimized. Future technical improvements for imaging perforating arteries or high-field systems will reveal the relationship of plaque and infarctions.

Third, the relationships among signal pattern of high-resolution magnetic resonance imaging, findings of magnetic resonance angiography, clinical symptoms, and characteristics of the plaques including thickness and distributions, and vulnerability, remain unclear, although cumulative evidences indicate intracranial plaque imaging allows characterization of plaques *in vivo*.

3. Conclusions

High-resolution magnetic resonance imaging can identify plaques on the walls of basilar artery or middle cerebral artery. This technique compensates the limitation of magnetic resonance angiography. However, further studies are needed to evaluate the limitations as described above. Besides these limitations, we consider that high-resolution magnetic resonance imaging is promising for the direct identification of intracranial arterial plaques and for the accurate estimation of the pathogenesis of the infarction, which will have an impact on the treatment strategy.

Prospective studies or long term follow up studies are needed to evaluate the accuracy and reproducibility.

4. References

Adams, HP Jr.; Bendixen, BH.; Kappelle, LJ.; Biller, J.; Love, BB.; Gordon, DL. & Marsh, EE 3rd. (1993). Classification of subtype of acute ischemic stroke. Definitions for use in a multicenter clinical trial. *Stroke,* Vol.24, No.1, (January 1993), pp. 35-41, ISSN 0039-2499

Arenillas, JF. (2011). Intracranial atherosclerosis: current concepts. *Stroke,* Vol.42, No.1 supplemental, (January 2011), pp. S20-S23, ISSN 1524-4628

Bassetti, C.; Bogousslavsky, J.; Barth, A. & Regli, F. (1996). Isolated infarcts of the pons. *Neurology,* Vol.46, No.1, (January 1996), pp. 165-175, ISSN 0028-3878

Cai, JM.; Hatsukami, TS.; Ferguson, MS.; Small, R.; Polissar, NL. & Yuan, C. (2002). Classification of human carotid atherosclerotic lesions with in vivo multicontrast magnetic resonance imaging. *Circulation,* Vol.106, No.11, (September 2002), pp. 1368-1373, ISSN 1524-4539

Chen, XY.; Wong, KS.; Lam, WW.; Zhao, HL. & Ng, HK. (2008). Middle cerebral artery atherosclerosis: histological comparison between plaques associated with and not associated with infarct in a postmortem study. *Cerebrovascular diseases,* Vol.25, No.1-2, (2008), pp. 74-80, ISSN 1421-9786

Cho, AH.; Kang, DW.; Kwon, SU. & Kim, JS. (2007). Is 15 mm size criterion for lacunar infarction still valid? A study on strictly subcortical middle cerebral artery territory infarction using diffusion-weighted MRI. *Cerebrovascular Diseases*, Vol.23, No.1, (2007), pp. 14-19, ISSN 1015-9770

Donnan, GA.; Bladin, PF.; Berkovic SF.; Longley, WA. & Saling, MM. (1991). The stroke syndrome of striatocapsular infarction. *Brain*, Vol.114 (Pt 1A), (February 1991), pp. 51-70, ISSN 0006-8950

Feyad, ZA. & Fuster, V. (2000). Characterization of atherosclerotic plaques by magnetic resonance imaging. *Annals of the New York Academy of Sciences*, Vol.902, (May 2000), pp. 173-186, ISSN 0077-8923

Fisher, CM. (1965). Lacunes: small, deep cerebral infarcts. *Neurology*, Vol.15, (August 1965), pp. 774-784, ISSN 0028-3878

Fisher, CM. & Caplan, LR. (1971). Basilar artery branch occlusion: a cause of pontine infarction. *Neurology*, Vol.21, No.9, (September 1971), pp. 900-905, ISSN 0028-3878

Fisher, CM. (1977). Bilateral occlusion of basilar artery branches. *Journal of Neurology, Neurosurgery, and Psychiatry*, Vol.40, No.12, (December 1977), pp. 1182-1189, ISSN 0022-3050

Fisher, CM. (1982). Lacunar strokes and infarcts: a review. *Neurology*, Vol.32, No.8, (August 1982), pp. 871-876, ISSN 0028-3878

Glagov, S.; Weisenberg, E.; Zarins, CK.; Stankunavicius, R. & Kolettis, GJ. (1987). Compensatory enlargement of human atherosclerotic coronary arteries. *The New England Journal of Medicine*, Vol.316, (May 1987), pp. 1371-1375, ISSN 0028-4793

Gorelick, PB.; Wong, KS.; Bae, HJ. & Pandey, DK. (2008). Large artery intracranial occlusive disease: a large worldwide burden but a relatively neglected frontier. *Stroke*, Vol.39, No.8, (August 2008), pp. 2396-2399, ISSN 1524-4628

Honda, M.; Kitagawa, N.; Tsutsumi, K.; Nagata, I.; Morikawa, M. & Hayashi, T. (2006). High-resolution magnetic resonance imaging for detection of carotid plaques. *Neurosurgery*, Vol.58, No.2, (February 2006), pp. 338-346, ISSN 1524-4040

Kern, R.; Steinke, W.; Daffertshofer, M.; Prager, R. & Hennerici M. (2005). Stroke recurrences in patients with symptomatic vs asymptomatic middle cerebral artery disease. *Neurology*, Vol.65, No.6, (September 2005), pp. 859-864, ISSN 1526-632X

Kim, JT.; Yoo, SH.; Kwon, JH.; Kwon, SU. & Kim, JS. (2006). Subtyping of ischemic stroke based on vascular imaging: analysis of 1167 acute, consecutive patients. *Journal of Clinical Neurology*, Vol.2, No.4, (December 2006), pp. 225-230, ISSN 2005-3013

Klein, IF.; Lavallëe, PC.; Schouman-Claeys, E. & Amarenco, P. (2005). High-resolution MRI identifies basilar artery plaques in paramedian pontine infarct. *Neurology*, Vol.64, No.3, (February 2005), pp. 551-552, ISSN 1526-632X

Klein, IF.; Lavallëe, PC.; Touboul, PJ.; Schouman-Claeys, E. & Amarenco, P. (2006). Middle cerebral artery plaque imaging by high-resolution MRI. *Neurology*, Vol.67, No.2, (July 2006), pp. 327-329, ISSN 1526-632X

Klein, IF.; Lavallëe, PC.; Mazighi, M.; Schouman-Claeys, E.; Labreuche, J. & Amarenco, P. (2010). Basilar artery atherosclerotic plaques in paramedian and lacunar pontine infarctions: a high-resolution MRI study. *Stroke*, Vol.41, No.7, (July 2010), pp. 1405-1409, ISSN 1524-4628

Kumral, E.; Bayülkem, G. & Evyapan, D. (2002). Clinical spectrum of pontine infarction. Clinical-MRI correlations. *Journal of Neurology*, Vol.249, No.12, (December 2002), pp. 1659-1670, ISSN 0340-5354

Li, ML.; Xu, WH.; Song, L.; Feng, F.; You, H.; Ni, J.; Gao, S.; Cui, LY. & Jin, ZY. (2009). Atherosclerosis of middle cerebral artery: evaluation with high-resolution MR imaging at 3T. *Atherosclerosis*, Vol.205, No.2, (June 2009), pp. 447-452, ISSN 1879-1484

Meyers, PM.; Schumacher, HC.; Gray, WA.; Fifi, J.; Gaudet, JG.; Heyer, EJ. & Chong, JY. (2009). Intravascular ultrasound of symptomatic intracranial stenosis demonstrates atherosclerotic plaque with intraplaque hemorrhage: a case report. *Journal of Neuroimaging,* Vol.19, No.3, (July 2009), pp. 266-270, ISSN 1552-6569

Niizuma, K.; Shimizu, H.; Takada, S. & Tominaga, T. (2008). Middle cerebral artery plaque imaging using 3-Tesla high-resolution MRI. *Journal of Clinical Neuroscience,* Vol.15, No.10, (October 2008), pp. 1137-1141, ISSN 0967-5868

Ryu, CW.; Jahng, GH.; Kim, EJ.; Choi, WS. & Yang, DM. (2009). High resolution wall and lumen MRI of the middle cerebral arteries at 3 tesla. *Cerebrovascular diseases,* Vol.27, No.5, (2009), pp. 433-442, ISSN 1421-9786

Shinnar, M.; Fallon, JT.; Wehrli, S.; Levin, M.; Dalmacy, D.; Fayad, ZA.; Badimon, JJ.; Harrington, M.; Harrington, E. & Fuster, V. (1999). The diagnostic accuracy of ex vivo MRI for human atherosclerotic plaque characterization. *Arteriosclerosis, thrombosis, and vascular biology,* Vol.19, No.11 (November 1999), pp. 2756-2761, ISSN 1079-5642

Swartz, RH.; Bhuta, SS.; Farb, RI.; Agid, R.; Willinsky, RA.; Terbruge, KG.; Butany, J.; Wasserman, BA.; Johnstone, DM.; Silver, FL. & Mikulis, DJ. (2009). Intracranial arterial wall imaging using high-resolution 3-tesla contrast-enhanced MRI. *Neurology,* Vol.72, No.7, (February 2009), pp. 627-634, ISSN 1526-632X

Toussaint, JF.; LaMuraglia, GM.; Southern, JF.; Fuster, V. & Kantor, HL. (1996). Magnetic resonance images lipid, fibrous, calcified, hemorrhagic, and thrombotic components of human atherosclerosis in vivo. *Circulation,* Vol.94, No.5, (September 1996), pp. 932–938, ISSN 0009-7322

Turan, TN.; Bonilha, L.; Morgan, PS.; Adams, RJ. & Chimowitz, MI. (2011). Intraplaque heorrhage in symptomatic intracranial atherosclerotic disease. *Journal of Neuroimaging,* Vol.21, No.2, (April 2011), pp. e159-e161, ISSN 1552-6569

Van der Kolk, AG.; Zwanenburg, JJ.; Brundel, M.; Biessels, GJ.; Visser, F.; Luijten, PR. & Hendrikse, J. (2011). Intracranial Vessel Wall Imaging at 7.0-T MRI. *Stroke,* Epub ahead of print, (July 2011), pp. e159-e161, ISSN 1524-4628

Wong, KS.; Huang, YN.; Gao, S.; Lam, WWM.; Chan, YL. & Kay, R. (1998). Intracranial stenosis in Chinese patients with acute stroke. *Neurology* Vol.50, No.3, (March 1998), pp. 812-813, ISSN 0028-3878

Xu, WH.; Li, ML.; Gao, S.; Ni, J.; Zhou, LX.; Yao, M.; Peng, B.; Feng, F.; Jin, ZY. & Cui, LY. (2010). In vivo high-resolution MR imaging of symptomatic and asymptomatic middle cerebral artery atherosclerotic stenosis. *Atherosclerosis,* Vol.212, No.2, (October 2010), pp. 507-411, ISSN 1879-1484

Yuan, C.; Mitsumori, LM.; Ferguson, MS.; Polissar, NL.; Echelard, D.; Ortiz, G.; Small, R.; Davies, JW.; Kerwin, WS. & Hatsukami, TS. (2001). In vivo accuracy of multispectral magnetic resonance imaging for identifying lipid-rich necrotic cores and intraplaque hemorrhage in advanced human carotid plaques. *Circulation,* Vol.104, No.17, (October 2001), pp. 2051-2056, ISSN 1524-4539

Yuan, C.; Kerwin, WS.; Ferguson, MS; Polissar, N.; Zhang, S.; Cai, J. & Hatsukami, TS. (2002a). Contrast-enhanced high resolution MRI for atherosclerotic carotid artery tissue characterization. *Journal of Magnetic Resonance Imaging,* Vol.15, No.1, (January 2002), pp. 62-67, ISSN 1053-1807

Yuan, C.; Miller, ZE.; Cai, J. & Hatsukami T. (2002b). Carotid atherosclerotic wall imaging by MRI. *Neuroimaging Clinics of North America,* Vol.12, No.3, (August 2002), pp. 391-401, ISSN 1052-5149

4

Intracranial Atherosclerotic Stroke - Hemodynamic Features and Role of MR Angiography

Suk Jae Kim and Oh Young Bang
Department of Neurology, Samsung Medical Center
Sungkyunkwan University, Seoul,
South Korea

1. Introduction

Intracranial atherosclerotic stroke (ICAS) is responsible for ischemic stroke in 10~33%.[1-3] ICAS occurs in association with various stroke mechanisms, such as in situ thrombotic occlusion, artery-to-artery embolism, hemodynamic insufficiency, and branch occlusion.[4] Various radiologic stroke patterns are associated with ICAS, from single and small subcortical perforator infarctions to multiple cortical infarctions [Figure 1].[5,6]

The characteristics of ICAS and the role of MRI and magnetic resonance angiography (MRA) are discussed herein.

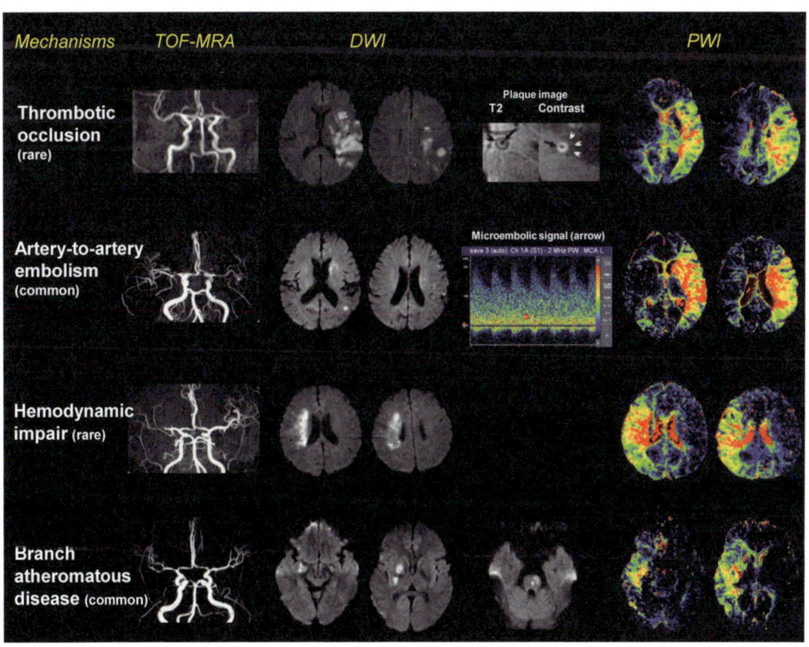

Fig. 1. Various mechanisms of stroke in patients with intracranial atherosclerosis.

2. Hemodynamic characteristics of ICAS

Despite of the diversity in stroke mechanisms of ICAS, ICAS has unique hemodynamics features compared to other stroke subtypes.

2.1 Pre-stroke hemodynamic status in patients with intracranial atherosclerosis

The balance of occlusion and collaterals determines the hemodynamic circumstance or blood flow changes that challenge the brain. Depending on the time course, such changes may have radically discrepant effects. Collateral circulation is a potent determinant of recurrent stroke risk in symptomatic ICAS, demonstrating a protective role with severe stenoses and identifying more unstable milder stenosis.[7] In addition, there are increasing evidences that ischemic preconditioning can induce tolerance by raising the threshold of tissue vulnerability in human brain.[8-10] Although ischemic brain injuries resulting from focal decrease in perfusion cause ischemic brain damage, patients with preceding less severe ischemic stimuli (i.e. transient ischemic attacks) showed less likely to have stroke and more likely to have good outcome after stroke.[8, 11] Longstanding hemodynamic compromise which was frequently observed in intracranial atherosclerosis may elicit collateral development and preconditioning to adapt to recurrent ischemia.[12] Thus, it is conceivable that patients with intracranial atherosclerosis may be 'prepared' and 'preconditioned' for the risk of subsequent stroke.

2.2 Hemodynamic feature in patients with ICAS

The most common techniques for imaging the ischemic penumbra in acute ischemic patients are (a) combined diffusion-weighted imaging (DWI) and perfusion-weighted imaging (PWI) and (b) combined DWI and MRA.[13-15] ICAS had a typical PWI-DWI (a large mismatch region but less severe hypoperfusion) and MRA-DWI mismatch profiles (a stenosis or occlusion of large intracranial vessels but a small core region), which have been reported to be associated with favorable outcomes after recanalization therapy.[16, 17] The differences in PWI-DWI and MRA-DWI mismatch profiles between ICAS and other stroke mechanisms may be related to differences in pretreatment collateral flow status [FIGURE 2].[17] Moreover, patients with ICAS had increased CBV when compared to patients with cardioembolic stroke.[18] Patients with ICAS had a good collateral grade than those with other subtypes.[17, 19, 20]

2.3 Stroke evolution, outcomes and recurrence after ICAS

There were two types of stroke evolution had different pathophysiological mechanisms.[21] Specifically, the large mild perfusion delay was associated with new lesions, whereas the large initial DWI lesions and a severe perfusion delay were associated with lesion growth.[21] Because patients with ICAS had relatively mild perfusion delay in their pretreatment MRI that were related to mostly multiple and small recurrent lesions, they may had minimal infarct growth [Figure 2].[16] Similarly, ICAS as a stroke mechanism resulted in favorable clinical outcomes. Benign pretreatment MR profiles which were associated with good collaterals of ICAS patients may explain these results.[16]

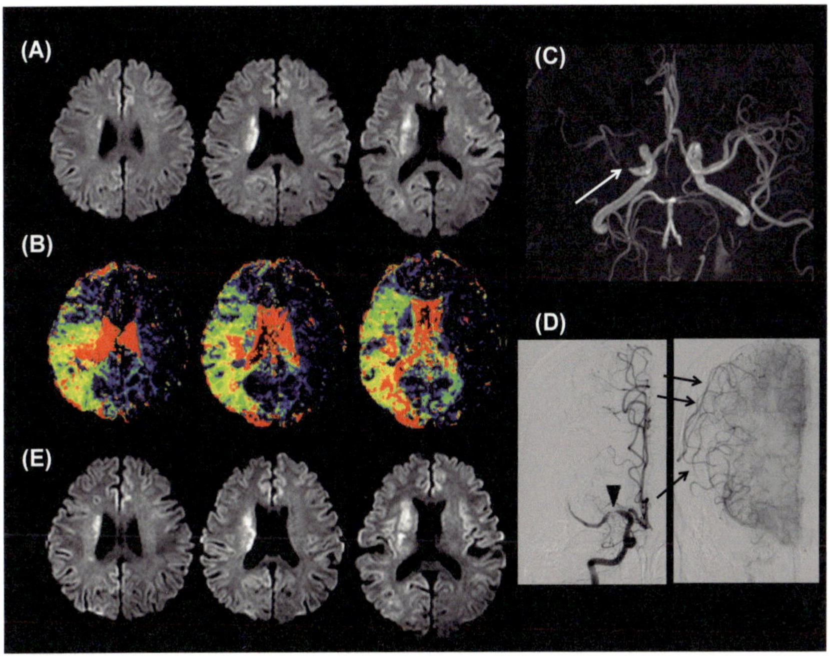

Fig. 2. Typical examples of intracranial atherosclerotic stroke. Initial MR shows typical PWI (B)-DWI (A) (a large salvageable area but less severe hypoperfusion) and MRA (C)-DWI (A) (a severe stenosis of right middle cerebral artery (white arrow) but a small core region). Digital subtraction angiography (D) demonstrates a severe stenosis in the same location (arrow head, arterial phase) and adequate leptomeningeal collateral flow from right anterior cerebral artery (black arrows, capillary phase). Follow-up DWI (E) reveals minimal infarct growth.

On the contrary, recurrent ischemic lesions during the first week after the onset of stroke in ICAS are relatively frequent compared to other stoke subtypes.[22] In clinical aspects, many patients with ICAS have recurrent cerebral ischemic events despite standard medical therapy with antiplatelet agents or oral anticoagulants.[23] The pattern of recurrence differed between intracranial and extracranial atherosclerotic stroke.[22, 24] Unlike the patients with carotid atherosclerosis who were unpredictable with respect to the site of recurrence and degree of preexisting stenosis, patients with ICAS usually recurred within the same territory as the index stroke which was associated with progression of stenosis.[5, 22, 24, 25] Collateral circulation is a potent determinant of recurrent stroke risk in symptomatic ICAS, demonstrating a protective role with severe stenoses and identifying more unstable milder stenosis.[7]

3. Vascular imaging in patients with ICAS

3.1 Vascular studies for luminal imaging

Digital subtraction angiography (DSA) is the current gold standard for the diagnosis of intracranial atherosclerosis. However, DSA is invasive and carries the risk of stroke. Along with transcranial Doppler (TCD) and computed tomographic angiography (CTA), MRA is less invasive techniques and has emerged as a more popular modality for visualization of intracranial vessels [Figure 3].

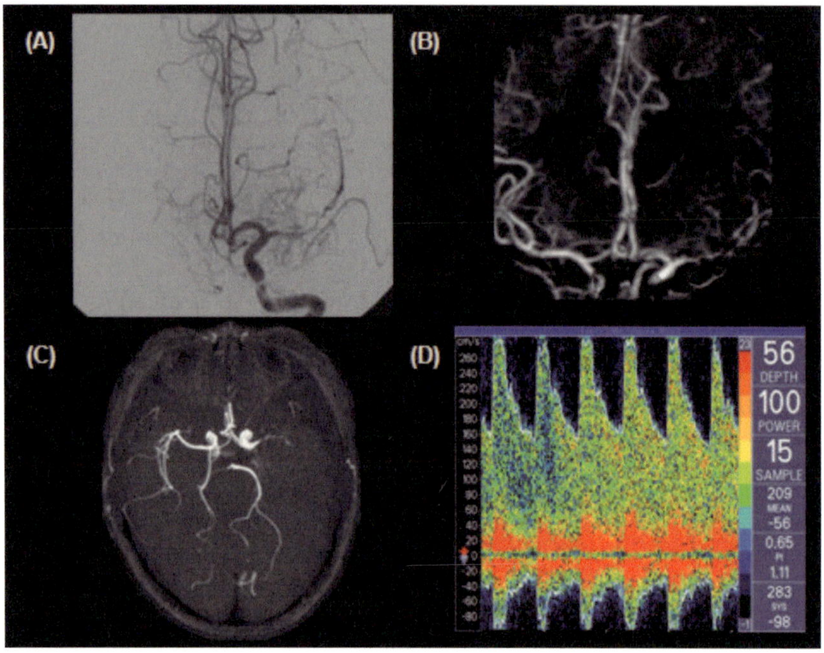

Fig. 3. A patient with intracranial stenosis on the left proximal middle cerebral artery. (A) DSA, (B) CTA, (C) TOF MRA, and (D) TCD findings.

Two MRA techniques used to detect intracranial stenosis are the 3D time-of-flight (TOF) MRA and contrast-enhanced MRA (CE-MRA). The Stroke Outcomes and Neuroimaging of Intracranial Atherosclerosis (SONIA) trial compared the accuracy of TOF MRA with DSA. SONIA demonstrated that TOF MRA have a good negative predictive value (89-93%) for excluding the presence of 50 to 99% intracranial atherosclerotic stenosis but relatively low positive predictive value (54-65%).[26, 27] CE-MRA is less studies for intracranial vessels because of technical issues. It has been thought that CE-MRA can lessen the problem of overestimation of the length and degree of stenosis, a common obstacle with 3D-TOF MRA by decreased dependence of flow signal intensity and T1 shortening effects of fat and calcium.[28, 29] However, recent studies suggested that TOF MRA provides comparable diagnostic performance with CE-MRA for intracranial stenosis with development of various TOF MRA sequence.[30, 31]

Recent advances in MRI techniques enable visualization of small perforating vessels originated from large intracranial arteries [Figure 4 D].[32] The Warfarin-Aspirin Symptomatic Intracranial Disease (WASID) trial investigators showed that the degree of stenosis (the presence of severe stenosis of ≥70%) was associated with subsequent ischemic stroke in the territory of the stenotic artery.[33] On the contrary, not only stenosis of severe degree but also stenosis of a milder degree on the symptomatic vessels should be taken into account, especially in patients with deep infarcts (branch occlusive disease). Physicians may consider a mild degree of stenosis to be irrelevant. However, large intracranial arteries have many deep perforators, and mild stenosis may occlude these deep perforators' orifices, resulting in stroke in the absence of plaque rupture or platelet activation. A follow-up study of patients with various subtypes of ischemic stroke demonstrated that, in patients with diagnoses of lacunar stroke at the time of their index strokes, physicians often found intracranial stenoses upon these patients' recurrences.[34]

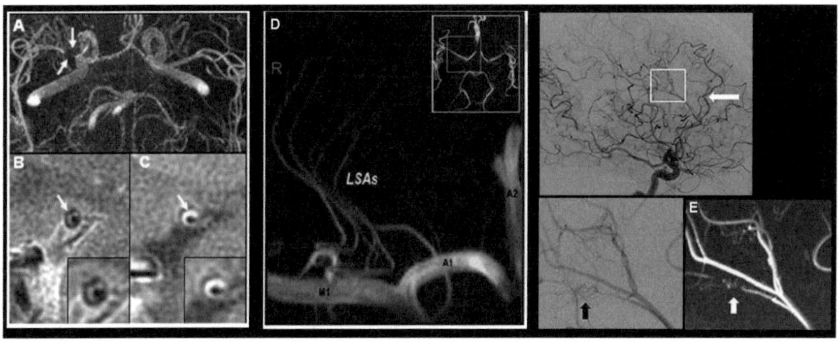

Fig. 4. Application of high resolution MRI. Contrast-enhanced MRI for plaque image (A-C), and 7-tesla MRA for small perforating arteries (D) and pial branches of leptomeningeal collaterals (E).

3.2 MRI for wall/plaque image

Patients with ICAS often have tandem lesions. Based on MRA, 65 out of 238 patients (27.3%) had coexistent asymptomatic intracranial stenosis. During a mean follow-up period of 1.8 years, 5 ischemic strokes (5.9%) occurred in the asymptomatic intracranial atherosclerotic stenosis territory (risk at 1 year=3.5%).[35] Thus, it is important to differentiate 'high-risk' stenosis and so called 'stable' (low-risk) stenosis.

There has been a growing body of interest in the role of MRI for imaging the vessel wall or the plaque. Autopsy series observed atherosclerotic plaques in intracranial vessels of 45.5-62.5% of subjects.[36,37] High-resolution MRI could provide the information on the presence and the volume of plaque.[38, 39] Plaque was clearly identified as plaque enhancement after gadolinium injection [Figure 4 A~C].[39]

MRI for plaque imaging is a potentially promising tool that can be used in clinical practice for patients with ICAS. First, this can be useful in evaluating the mechanisms of stroke, i.e. demonstrating the presence of intracranial plaque in patients with cryptogenic stroke. High-resolution MRI to determine the presence of plaque revealed that MRI detects basilar artery plaques in 42% of patients with pontine infarctions and normal basilar angiograms.[38] Second, this technique can help physician to identify the vulnerable plaque in the intracranial vessels. A recent study showed that all patients with ICAS have eccentric enhancing plaques when imaging is performed within weeks to months of cerebral infarcts within the artery territory, but none of asymptomatic plaques had enhancement.[40] Moreover, remodeling mode of intracranial atherosclerosis can be identified using high-resolution MRI. It has been well known that atherosclerotic narrowing of arterial lumen is not a simple consequence of enlargement of atherosclerotic burden.[41] Recent investigations with patients with intracranial atherosclerotic stenosis revealed that some compensatory enlargement of vessels (positive remodeling) which is associated with more lipid-rich plaques[42, 43] was more frequently observed in symptomatic patients compared with asymptomatic ones.[44, 45] Lastly, risk factors for the presence of intracranial plaque have been reported[36] and several drug therapies (i.e. statin) could modify plaque stability. In addition, the effects of such therapeutic intervention could be monitored using high-resolution MRI.

3.3 Collateral image

MRA can evaluate the cerebral collateral circulation in the circle of Willis. With phase contrast MRA, flow direction information can be obtained by the phase changes in blood water protons in the different arterial segments of the circle of Willis.[46] Although MRA have moderate to good diagnostic performance for the presence of collateral flow via the anterior circle of Willis, MRA tends to underestimate the presence of collateral flow with respect to the posterior communicating artery. Compared to conventional angiography which is considered as a gold standard for the assessment of collaterals, MRA collateral flow measurements via the anterior part of the circle of Willis yielded a sensitivity, specificity, positive predictive value, negative predictive value and accuracy of 83%, 77%, 78%, 82% and 80%, respectively. On the other hand, MRA collateral flow measurements via the posterior communicating artery yielded a sensitivity, specificity, positive predictive value, negative predictive value and accuracy of 33%, 88%, 89%, 31% and 47%, respectively.[47-49] Recently, vessel-encoded arterial spin labeling technique was developed to assess collateral circulations.[50-52]

Beside the collateral circulation via the circle of Willis, leptomeningeal collaterals also play an important role in patients with ICAS. The leptomeningeal collateral can be visualized using a dedicated MRI method (subtracting the image of the first movement map).[53] Beside the vessel images, various MRI parameters can indirectly reflect the collateral status, e.g. DWI, PWI, and FLAIR. We found that, compared to the large cortical DWI pattern, the deep-infarcts pattern exhibited less severe hypoperfusion related to good collateral flows.[54] In addition, distal hyperintense vessels on fluid-attenuated inversion recovery image likely represent excessively slow flow induced by retrograde collateral flow distal to the occlusion of a proximal artery, and may be associated with leptomeningeal collaterals and response to thrombolysis.[55, 56] A recent study using 7-tesla MRI directly visualized the pial branches, indicating the possibility of assessment of leptomeningeal collaterals with high-resolution MRA [Figure 4 E].[57]

4. Conclusion

Patients with ICAS often received the same treatment as those with extracranial carotid atherosclerosis. However, there are accumulating evidences that hemodynamic features as well as stroke mechanisms may differ between ICAS and other stroke subtypes.[24, 58, 59] Using MRI techniques to understanding pathophysiologies, hemodynamic status, and vascular pathology (via both luminal and wall imaging) will allow the future development of rational stroke therapies for patients with ICAS.

5. References

[1] Sacco RL, Kargman DE, Gu Q, Zamanillo MC. Race-ethnicity and determinants of intracranial atherosclerotic cerebral infarction. The northern manhattan stroke study. *Stroke*. 1995;26:14-20

[2] Wityk RJ, Lehman D, Klag M, Coresh J, Ahn H, Litt B. Race and sex differences in the distribution of cerebral atherosclerosis. *Stroke*. 1996;27:1974-1980

[3] Wong KS, Huang YN, Gao S, Lam WW, Chan YL, Kay R. Intracranial stenosis in chinese patients with acute stroke. *Neurology*. 1998;50:812-813

[4] Kim JS CL, Wong KS, eds. *Intracranial atherosclerosis*. Wiley-Blackwell: John Wiley and Sons, Ltd.; 2008.

[5] Wong KS, Gao S, Chan YL, Hansberg T, Lam WW, Droste DW, Kay R, Ringelstein EB. Mechanisms of acute cerebral infarctions in patients with middle cerebral artery stenosis: A diffusion-weighted imaging and microemboli monitoring study. *Ann Neurol*. 2002;52:74-81

[6] Bang OY, Heo JH, Kim JY, Park JH, Huh K. Middle cerebral artery stenosis is a major clinical determinant in striatocapsular small, deep infarction. *Arch Neurol*. 2002;59:259-263

[7] Liebeskind DS, Cotsonis GA, Saver JL, Lynn MJ, Turan TN, Cloft HJ, Chimowitz MI. Collaterals dramatically alter stroke risk in intracranial atherosclerosis. *Ann Neurol*. 2011;69:963-974

[8] Dirnagl U, Becker K, Meisel A. Preconditioning and tolerance against cerebral ischaemia: From experimental strategies to clinical use. *Lancet Neurol*. 2009;8:398-412

[9] Gidday JM. Cerebral preconditioning and ischaemic tolerance. *Nat Rev Neurosci*. 2006;7:437-448

[10] Kharbanda RK, Nielsen TT, Redington AN. Translation of remote ischaemic preconditioning into clinical practice. *Lancet*. 2009;374:1557-1565

[11] Wegener S, Gottschalk B, Jovanovic V, Knab R, Fiebach JB, Schellinger PD, Kucinski T, Jungehulsing GJ, Brunecker P, Muller B, Banasik A, Amberger N, Wernecke KD, Siebler M, Rother J, Villringer A, Weih M. Transient ischemic attacks before ischemic stroke: Preconditioning the human brain? A multicenter magnetic resonance imaging study. *Stroke*. 2004;35:616-621

[12] Liebeskind DS. Imaging the future of stroke: I. Ischemia. *Ann Neurol*. 2009;66:574-590

[13] Albers GW, Thijs VN, Wechsler L, Kemp S, Schlaug G, Skalabrin E, Bammer R, Kakuda W, Lansberg MG, Shuaib A, Coplin W, Hamilton S, Moseley M, Marks MP. Magnetic resonance imaging profiles predict clinical response to early reperfusion: The diffusion and perfusion imaging evaluation for understanding stroke evolution (defuse) study. *Ann Neurol*. 2006;60:508-517

[14] Bang OY. Multimodal mri for ischemic stroke: From acute therapy to preventive strategies. *J Clin Neurol*. 2009;5:107-119

[15] Lansberg MG, Thijs VN, Bammer R, Olivot JM, Marks MP, Wechsler LR, Kemp S, Albers GW. The mra-dwi mismatch identifies patients with stroke who are likely to benefit from reperfusion. *Stroke*. 2008;39:2491-2496

[16] Kim SJ, Ryoo S, Kim GM, Chung CS, Lee KH, Bang OY. Clinical and radiological outcomes after intracranial atherosclerotic stroke: A comprehensive approach comparing stroke subtypes. *Cerebrovasc Dis*. 2011;31:427-434

[17] Kim SJ, Seok JM, Bang OY, Kim GM, Kim KH, Jeon P, Chung CS, Lee KH, Alger JR, Liebeskind DS. Mr mismatch profiles in patients with intracranial atherosclerotic stroke: A comprehensive approach comparing stroke subtypes. *J Cereb Blood Flow Metab*. 2009;29:1138-1145

[18] Liebeskind DS, Alger JR, Kim GM, Sanossian N, Chung CS, Lee KH, Bang OY. Collateral perfusion and cerebral blood volume diminish infarct core and penumbra in acute ischemic stroke due to intracranial atherosclerosis. *Stroke.* 2009;40:e119
[19] Choi JW, Kim JK, Choi BS, Lim HK, Kim SJ, Kim JS, Suh DC. Angiographic pattern of symptomatic severe m1 stenosis: Comparison with presenting symptoms, infarct patterns, perfusion status, and outcome after recanalization. *Cerebrovasc Dis.* 2010;29:297-303
[20] Liebeskind DS, Cotsonis GA, Saver JL, Lynn MJ, Cloft HJ, Chimowitz MI. Collateral circulation in symptomatic intracranial atherosclerosis. *J Cereb Blood Flow Metab.* 2011;31:1293-1301
[21] Bang OY, Kim GM, Chung CS, Kim SJ, Kim KH, Jeon P, Saver JL, Liebeskind DS, Lee KH. Differential pathophysiological mechanisms of stroke evolution between new lesions and lesion growth: Perfusion-weighted imaging study. *Cerebrovasc Dis.* 2010;29:328-335
[22] Kang DW, Kwon SU, Yoo SH, Kwon KY, Choi CG, Kim SJ, Koh JY, Kim JS. Early recurrent ischemic lesions on diffusion-weighted imaging in symptomatic intracranial atherosclerosis. *Arch Neurol.* 2007;64:50-54
[23] Chimowitz MI, Lynn MJ, Howlett-Smith H, Stern BJ, Hertzberg VS, Frankel MR, Levine SR, Chaturvedi S, Kasner SE, Benesch CG, Sila CA, Jovin TG, Romano JG. Comparison of warfarin and aspirin for symptomatic intracranial arterial stenosis. *N Engl J Med.* 2005;352:1305-1316
[24] Shin DH, Lee PH, Bang OY. Mechanisms of recurrence in subtypes of ischemic stroke: A hospital-based follow-up study. *Arch Neurol.* 2005;62:1232-1237
[25] Wong KS, Li H, Lam WW, Chan YL, Kay R. Progression of middle cerebral artery occlusive disease and its relationship with further vascular events after stroke. *Stroke.* 2002;33:532-536
[26] Feldmann E, Wilterdink JL, Kosinski A, Lynn M, Chimowitz MI, Sarafin J, Smith HH, Nichols F, Rogg J, Cloft HJ, Wechsler L, Saver J, Levine SR, Tegeler C, Adams R, Sloan M. The stroke outcomes and neuroimaging of intracranial atherosclerosis (sonia) trial. *Neurology.* 2007;68:2099-2106
[27] Qureshi AI, Feldmann E, Gomez CR, Johnston SC, Kasner SE, Quick DC, Rasmussen PA, Suri MF, Taylor RA, Zaidat OO. Intracranial atherosclerotic disease: An update. *Ann Neurol.* 2009;66:730-738
[28] Jung HW, Chang KH, Choi DS, Han MH, Han MC. Contrast-enhanced mr angiography for the diagnosis of intracranial vascular disease: Optimal dose of gadopentetate dimeglumine. *AJR Am J Roentgenol.* 1995;165:1251-1255
[29] Bash S, Villablanca JP, Jahan R, Duckwiler G, Tillis M, Kidwell C, Saver J, Sayre J. Intracranial vascular stenosis and occlusive disease: Evaluation with ct angiography, mr angiography, and digital subtraction angiography. *AJNR Am J Neuroradiol.* 2005;26:1012-1021
[30] Choi J, Lim, SM, Kim, Y. Comparison of 3d tof mra with contrast enhanced mra in intracranial atherosclerotic occlusive disease. *J Korean Soc Radiol.* 2011;64:203-211
[31] Babiarz LS, Romero JM, Murphy EK, Brobeck B, Schaefer PW, Gonzalez RG, Lev MH. Contrast-enhanced mr angiography is not more accurate than unenhanced 2d time-

of-flight mr angiography for determining > or = 70% internal carotid artery stenosis. *AJNR Am J Neuroradiol*. 2009;30:761-768

[32] Cho ZH, Kang CK, Han JY, Kim SH, Kim KN, Hong SM, Park CW, Kim YB. Observation of the lenticulostriate arteries in the human brain in vivo using 7.0t mr angiography. *Stroke*. 2008;39:1604-1606

[33] Kasner SE, Chimowitz MI, Lynn MJ, Howlett-Smith H, Stern BJ, Hertzberg VS, Frankel MR, Levine SR, Chaturvedi S, Benesch CG, Sila CA, Jovin TG, Romano JG, Cloft HJ. Predictors of ischemic stroke in the territory of a symptomatic intracranial arterial stenosis. *Circulation*. 2006;113:555-563

[34] Shin DH, Lee PH, Bang OY. Mechanisms of recurrence in subtypes of ischemic stroke: A hospital-based follow-up study. *Archives of neurology*. 2005;62:1232-1237

[35] Nahab F, Cotsonis G, Lynn M, Feldmann E, Chaturvedi S, Hemphill JC, Zweifler R, Johnston K, Bonovich D, Kasner S, Chimowitz M. Prevalence and prognosis of coexistent asymptomatic intracranial stenosis. *Stroke*. 2008;39:1039-1041

[36] Mazighi M, Labreuche J, Gongora-Rivera F, Duyckaerts C, Hauw JJ, Amarenco P. Autopsy prevalence of intracranial atherosclerosis in patients with fatal stroke. *Stroke*. 2008;39:1142-1147

[37] Chen XY, Wong KS, Lam WW, Zhao HL, Ng HK. Middle cerebral artery atherosclerosis: Histological comparison between plaques associated with and not associated with infarct in a postmortem study. *Cerebrovasc Dis*. 2008;25:74-80

[38] Klein IF, Lavallee PC, Mazighi M, Schouman-Claeys E, Labreuche J, Amarenco P. Basilar artery atherosclerotic plaques in paramedian and lacunar pontine infarctions: A high-resolution mri study. *Stroke*. 2010;41:1405-1409

[39] Klein IF, Lavallee PC, Touboul PJ, Schouman-Claeys E, Amarenco P. In vivo middle cerebral artery plaque imaging by high-resolution mri. *Neurology*. 2006;67:327-329

[40] Vergouwen MD, Silver FL, Mandell DM, Mikulis DJ, Swartz RH. Eccentric narrowing and enhancement of symptomatic middle cerebral artery stenoses in patients with recent ischemic stroke. *Arch Neurol*. 2011;68:338-342

[41] Glagov S, Weisenberg E, Zarins CK, Stankunavicius R, Kolettis GJ. Compensatory enlargement of human atherosclerotic coronary arteries. *N Engl J Med*. 1987;316:1371-1375

[42] Burke AP, Kolodgie FD, Farb A, Weber D, Virmani R. Morphological predictors of arterial remodeling in coronary atherosclerosis. *Circulation*. 2002;105:297-303

[43] Takeuchi H, Morino Y, Matsukage T, Masuda N, Kawamura Y, Kasai S, Hashida T, Fujibayashi D, Tanabe T, Ikari Y. Impact of vascular remodeling on the coronary plaque compositions: An investigation with in vivo tissue characterization using integrated backscatter-intravascular ultrasound. *Atherosclerosis*. 2009;202:476-482

[44] Ma N, Jiang WJ, Lou X, Ma L, Du B, Cai JF, Zhao TQ. Arterial remodeling of advanced basilar atherosclerosis: A 3-tesla mri study. *Neurology*. 2010;75:253-258

[45] Xu WH, Li ML, Gao S, Ni J, Zhou LX, Yao M, Peng B, Feng F, Jin ZY, Cui LY. In vivo high-resolution mr imaging of symptomatic and asymptomatic middle cerebral artery atherosclerotic stenosis. *Atherosclerosis*. 2010;212:507-511

[46] Sallustio F, Kern R, Gunther M, Szabo K, Griebe M, Meairs S, Hennerici M, Gass A. Assessment of intracranial collateral flow by using dynamic arterial spin labeling mra and transcranial color-coded duplex ultrasound. *Stroke*. 2008;39:1894-1897

[47] Patrux B, Laissy JP, Jouini S, Kawiecki W, Coty P, Thiebot J. Magnetic resonance angiography (mra) of the circle of willis: A prospective comparison with conventional angiography in 54 subjects. *Neuroradiology*. 1994;36:193-197

[48] Hartkamp MJ, van Der Grond J, van Everdingen KJ, Hillen B, Mali WP. Circle of willis collateral flow investigated by magnetic resonance angiography. *Stroke*. 1999;30:2671-2678

[49] Hendrikse J, Klijn CJ, van Huffelen AC, Kappelle LJ, van der Grond J. Diagnosing cerebral collateral flow patterns: Accuracy of non-invasive testing. *Cerebrovasc Dis*. 2008;25:430-437

[50] Chng SM, Petersen ET, Zimine I, Sitoh YY, Lim CC, Golay X. Territorial arterial spin labeling in the assessment of collateral circulation: Comparison with digital subtraction angiography. *Stroke*. 2008;39:3248-3254

[51] Kansagra AP, Wong EC. Quantitative assessment of mixed cerebral vascular territory supply with vessel encoded arterial spin labeling mri. *Stroke*. 2008;39:2980-2985

[52] Wu B, Wang X, Guo J, Xie S, Wong EC, Zhang J, Jiang X, Fang J. Collateral circulation imaging: Mr perfusion territory arterial spin-labeling at 3t. *AJNR Am J Neuroradiol*. 2008;29:1855-1860

[53] Christensen S, Calamante F, Hjort N, Wu O, Blankholm AD, Desmond P, Davis S, Ostergaard L. Inferring origin of vascular supply from tracer arrival timing patterns using bolus tracking mri. *J Magn Reson Imaging*. 2008;27:1371-1381

[54] Bang OY, Saver JL, Alger JR, Starkman S, Ovbiagele B, Liebeskind DS. Determinants of the distribution and severity of hypoperfusion in patients with ischemic stroke. *Neurology*. 2008;71:1804-1811

[55] Lee KY, Latour LL, Luby M, Hsia AW, Merino JG, Warach S. Distal hyperintense vessels on flair: An mri marker for collateral circulation in acute stroke? *Neurology*. 2009;72:1134-1139

[56] Liebeskind DS. Location, location, location: Angiography discerns early mr imaging vessel signs due to proximal arterial occlusion and distal collateral flow. *AJNR Am J Neuroradiol*. 2005;26:2432-2433; author reply 2433-2434

[57] Song HS, Kang CK, Kim JS, Park CA, Kim YB, Lee DH, Kang DW, Kwon SU, Cho ZH. Assessment of pial branches using 7-tesla mri in cerebral arterial disease. *Cerebrovasc Dis*. 2010;29:410

[58] Bang OY, Kim JW, Lee JH, Lee MA, Lee PH, Joo IS, Huh K. Association of the metabolic syndrome with intracranial atherosclerotic stroke. *Neurology*. 2005;65:296-298

[59] Bang OY, Lee PH, Yoon SR, Lee MA, Joo IS, Huh K. Inflammatory markers, rather than conventional risk factors, are different between carotid and mca atherosclerosis. *J Neurol Neurosurg Psychiatry*. 2005;76:1128-1134

5

Clinical Applications of Quantitative MRA in Neurovascular Practice

Aaron R. Ducoffe[1], Angelos A. Konstas[2],
John Pile-Spellman[3] and Jonathan L. Brisman[3]
[1]*Emory University School of Medicine*
[2]*University of California, Los Angeles*
[3]*Neurological Surgery, P.C.*
USA

1. Introduction

QMRA, quantitative magnetic resonance angiography, is currently the only non-invasive modality with which to quantify blood flow in the human vasculature. Dr. Fady Charbel, a vascular neurosurgeon at the University of Chicago, spearheaded the application of this technology to the cerebrovascular system. Knowledge and experience garnered through years of research by Dr. Charbel and others on computer modeling and circulatory fluid dynamics culminated in the development of computer software referred to as non-invasive optimal vessel analysis (NOVA) (Zhao et al., 2000). QMRA uses traditional time-of-flight and phase-contrast MRI to visualize extracranial and intracranial vascular anatomy and measure volumetric blood flow. VasSol Inc., through which the software is now commercially available, acquired pre-market FDA approval for the technology in 2002.

NOVA is currently in use at 24 centers throughout this country and in only six centers outside the United States. Just a few publications have appeared using this technology. Reports on NOVA have been published demonstrating its use as a decision-making tool for patients with vertebrobasilar ischemia (Amin-Hanjani et al., 2005), as a means to document vascular bypass patency (Amin-Hanjani et al., 2007), as a means to evaluate in-stent stenosis after intracranial stent placement (Prabhakaran et al., 2009), as a measure of successful embolization of Vein of Galen malformations (Langer et al., 2006b), as a means to determine whether patients will tolerate carotid occlusion (Charbel et al., 2004), as a means to study vertebrobasilar flow in patients with subclavian steal syndrome (Bauer et al., 2008), as a means to quantify blood volume from leptomeningeal collaterals in patients with anterior circulation stenoses (Ruland et al., 2008), as a means to quantify carotid blood flow changes after carotid endarterectomy and carotid angioplasty and stenting for atherosclerotic disease (Ghogawala et al., 2008) and as a means to understand a difficult case of hemispheric ischemia and subclavian stenosis and plan treatment (Langer et al., 2006a). Most recently, we published on the reproducible use of NOVA to demonstrate arterial waveform changes both before and after a neurovascular intervention in ten patients (Brisman et al., 2011).

This chapter documents the use of NOVA for a cohort of 19 patients with a variety of cerebrovascular diseases. Nineteen cases treated over an 18-month period are discussed, 10 of whom had arterial waveform data previously reported (Brisman et al., 2011). The benefits, limits and potential pitfalls of the technology are evaluated.

2. Patients and methods

All NOVA procedures were performed on a 1.5 Tesla MRI. NOVA can study the intracranial, cervical and/or aortic vasculature, as well as the vascular system of other body parts such as the kidneys. Gadolinium is not required for NOVA, but would be given if it were deemed worthwhile for the MRA (which is always obtained as part of the NOVA test) or if an additional brain or spine MRI was performed that required it. On average, NOVA added 25-40 minutes to the MRI scan time, depending on technical experience and complexity of the case.

Retrospective review of all NOVA studies was approved by the IRB of the treating institution. Each NOVA was given one of three scores by the authors based on its perceived clinical utility as follows: CD (Clinical Decision-making) = NOVA results altered decision-making for the patient in a substantial way. This generally meant that a procedure was or was not offered to the patient based on NOVA results or that the type of procedure performed was decided based on NOVA; HP (Hypothesized Pathophysiology) = NOVA results were consistent with the clinical picture such that the authors felt that NOVA further supported the management strategy but the results did not alter treatment. This score also was given in situations where the NOVA findings had no bearing on decision-making but reflected what one would expect from the disease entity, i.e. a brain AVM showing increased flow in feeding arteries and draining veins, or an area of significant stenosis showing decreased flow; NUD (No Useful Data) = NOVA yielded data that was confusing or contrary to what is generally understood about a particular disease entity. The NUD score was also given in instances where there was no apparent alteration of flow that may have simply reflected the disease entity considered, i.e. NOVA results on a patient with a small intracranial aneurysm.

Note was also made of results for blood vessels separate from the region of interest that were abnormal with no ready explanation, which for simplicity we will call "false positive" data. Abnormal values were grouped into those that were 10-50 cc/min higher or lower than the expected normal baseline values and those that were 50 cc/min higher or lower than the expected normal values (Table 1). The distinction between "false positive" data, and data that would result in a NUD designation is that "false positive" values were typically recorded for blood vessels distinct from the region of pathologic interest. A patient with HP data for the region of interest, for example, might also have values for vessels that the were felt to be unrelated in a straightforward fashion to the region of interest and therefore while these specific values might be hard to interpret they did not necessarily affect the overall designation of the study.

3. Results

Twenty-Nine NOVA studies were performed over an 18 month period on 19 patients for a wide variety of cerebrovascular pathologies including vasospasm after aneurysmal SAH (1 patient), gamma knife radiosurgery of brain AVMs (3), carotid stenosis from fibromuscular dysplasia (2), high-flow (1) and low-flow bypass (1), angioplasty and stenting using the

Wingspan Stent (2), Neuroform-stenting and coiling of aneurysms (2), and conservatively treated atherosclerotic intracranial disease (2) (Table 1). Two patients with non-vascular pathology were also studied. In 13/19 (68%) patients an intervention was performed after the initial NOVA study; of those 10/13 (77%) had post-procedure repeat NOVA studies. NOVA was found to be CD in 4/19 patients (21%), HP in 12/19 (63%) and NUD in 3/19 (16%). The test was CD or HP in 10/10 cases in which NOVA was performed before and after an intervention. False positive values were found in 12/29 (41%) studies, nine of which had an abnormal value 50 cc/min less than or greater than normal.

Age/Sex	Pathology	QMRA BaL	Intervention	QMRA PP	QMRA Score	False Positive
61F	Paraclinoid Aneurysm	Normal	Stent/Coil	NA	NUD	BA↓↓84, LMCA↓99
63F	SAH/Acomm Aneurysm	RMCA↓↓62	Clipping "Triple H"	RMCA119	HP	
56F	Hydocephalus Colloid Cyst	Normal	VPS	NA	NUD	
72M	Carotid Stenosis	RICA↓117	CAS	NA	HP	
66F	Basilar Aneurysm Subclavian Stenosis	**LVA↓-30, BA↓↓74, LPCA↓29, RPCA40**	Subclavian Angioplasty/Stent Aneurysm Stent/Coil	LVA122, BA145, LPCA56, RPCA77	CD	**LCCA↓↓253 RCCA↓↓220 LACA↓↓33 LMCA↓91**
79F	Basilar Stenosis	BA↓40	None	NA	HP	LVA↓31 RVA↓68
62M (Case 2)	LCCA Occlusion	**LMCA↓65, LCCA↓↓0**	Subclavian/Carotid Bypass	Bypass 242, LICA↓164, LMCA 111	HP	**RCCA↓↓158** RCCA↓↓243 BA↓143
49F	LICA FMD	LCCA↓↓146, LICA↓↓63, RICA↑↑443, LACA↓↓-99, RACA↑↑188, LPCA↑112	None	NA	HP	
39F (Case 1)	R Temporal AVM	RCCA↑↑448, RPCA↑↑130, LTS 215, RTS 871, STS 542, BVR 405	GKR	RCCA↑↑397 SSS 343, LTS 487, RTS 661, STS 487, BVR 341	HP	
65F	Basilar Stenosis	BA↓↓18	None	NA	HP	
65F	Subfrontal AVM	LTS 132, RTS 573, STS 117, SAS 510	GKR	RCCA 271, SSS 402, LTS 102, RTS 354, STS 83	HP	
36F (Case 5)	RICA FMD	RCCA↓↓160, RICA↓↓74	RCAS	RICA 212, BA 143	HP	RACA↓↓29 LVA↑197
31F	R Parietal AVM	RMCA↑↑741, LACA↑238, SSS 724, STS 81, RTS 656, LTS 325	GKR	RMCA↑↑541, RICA↑↑457, LICA↑↑500, LACA↑↑249, RTS 605, LTS 424, SSS 738, STS 101, DV 30	HP	

Age/Sex	Pathology	QMRA BaL	Intervention	QMRA PP	QMRA Score	False Positive
70F	Meningioma Resection	LICA↓↓154, RICA↓↓132			NUD	BA↓↓114 RPCA↓36
63F	R TS Dural Fistula	Normal	None	NA	NUD	LICA↓↓168 RICA↓↓142 BA↓↓122
54F	RICA Occlusion	**RICA↓↓0, RCCA↓↓115, RMCA↓↓44, LACA↓↓-195, RACA↓↓-45, RPCA↑140, LMCA 206**	STA/MCA Bypass	RMCA↓↓27, RCCA↓↓146, LMCA 249, LACA-261, RACA-18, RPCA 108 (Normal)	HP	LVA↑206 LACA↓↓-261
52M (Case 3)	Multiple Sx. BL Vertebral Stenoses	**LVA↓↓26, RVA↓↓58, BA↓↓5**	VA/Stent	BA1↓40, LVA 179, RVA↓↓26	CD	RCCA↓288, LICA↓165, LACA↓40
55M	SAH/Pcomm Aneurysm	NA	Stent/Coil	Normal (X mos.)	NUD	
69M (Case 4)	Sx. Right Vertebral Stenosis	**RVA↓↓26, (BA157)**	VA/Stent	RVA 73, (BA 166)	HD	RACA↓41, RCCA↓287, LVA↑189, LACA↓↓-306, LICA↑↑366, LPCA↑115

Table 1. QMRA Cases: Key: False Positive = the results of NOVA had no simple explanation based on the pathology and could not be explained by the authors. Note: in instances where there was False Positives and two NOVA studies had been performed, one before and one after an intervention, boldface was used to clarify which study the data was from. BaL = baseline, PP = postprocedureless, BL = bilateral, NA = not available, ↓ or ↑= between 10-50ml/min outside normal expected QMRA values in the direction of the arrow, ↓↓ or ↑↑ = greater than 50ml/min beyond the normal expected QMRA values in the direction of the arrows, GKR = gamma knife radiosurgery, CAS = carotid angioplasty and stinting, Sx. = symptomatic.

4. Case illustrations

4.1 Case 1

The patient is a 39-year-old otherwise healthy woman who presented five years previously with headaches and was found to have a right medial temporal arteriovenous malformation. She was offered intervention at that time, including surgical excision, but because of the quoted risks of the procedure the patient declined. She more recently presented to medical attention when she developed an acute onset headache associated with nausea and lightheadedness. CT scan of the brain showed a small subarachnoid hemorrhage adjacent to the AVM. Angiography showed the lesion to be fed primarily from enlarged branches of the posterior communicating artery and posterior cerebral artery. Venous egress was deep to an enlarged basal vein of Rosenthal and then to a dominant right transverse sinus (TS) (Figure

1A). NOVA analysis showed increased flow in the carotid artery and posterior cerebral artery on the side of the lesion with high flow in the draining basal vein of Rosenthal and the right TS relative to the left (Figure 1B-E).

After consideration of different treatment strategies, the patient was treated with gamma knife radiosurgery. Six months later, the MRI appearance was without change. NOVA analysis, however, showed a decrease in the flow through the carotid artery on the right as well as a decrease in the flow through the right TS and draining basal vein (Figure 1F-G).

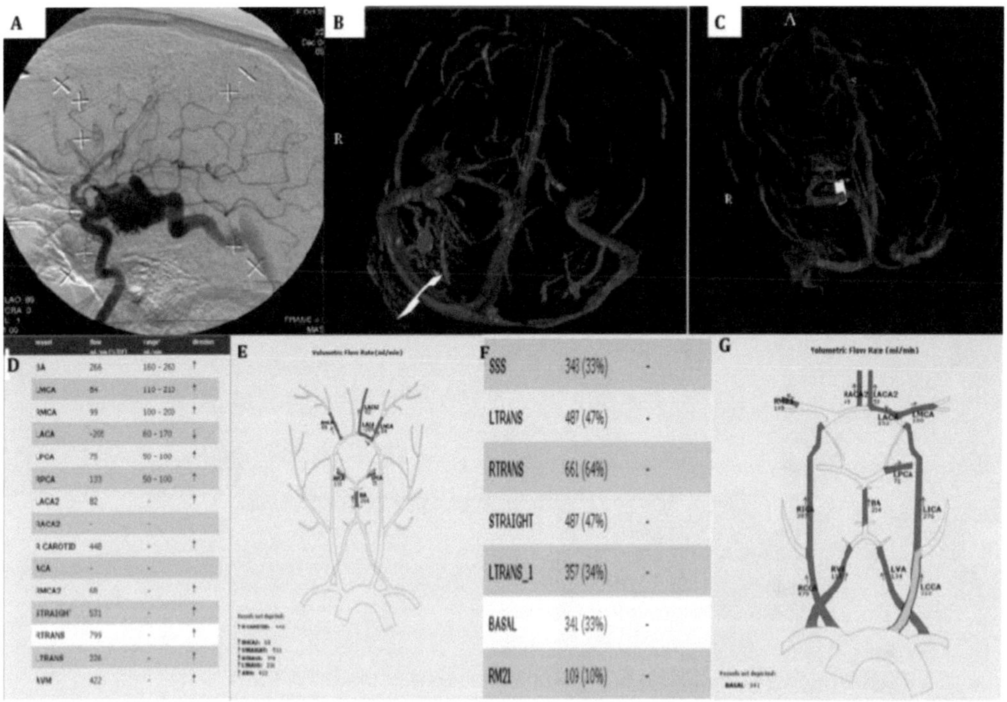

Fig. 1. Case 1 Images: A, Lateral angiogram, right internal carotid injection (postero-anterior view) shows a medio-temporal AVM nidus fed by the posterior communicator, its perforators and the posterior cerebral artery and its perforators and draining through the basal vein of Rosenthal to the deep venous system and ultimately to the transverse sinus. B, C, NOVA 3D surface rendering shows the AVM nidus with the yellow cursor demonstrating where the flow was measured in the right transverse sinus (B) and basal vein of Rosenthal (C). D,E, NOVA baseline table (D) and vessel map (E) pre-radiosurgery demonstrates abnormally increased flow in the right posterior cerebral artery (PCA) and internal carotid artery (ICA) with marked asymmetry of flow in the right transverse sinus compared with the left. Flow in the basal vein is denoted "AVM" and is also quantitated. F, G NOVA baseline table (F) and vessel map (G) six months post-radiosurgery shows marked decreased in flow in the basilar, right ICA, basal vein of Rosenthal and transverse sinus.

4.2 Case 2

This 62-year-old man presented to an outside facility with the acute onset of a right hemiparesis, affecting the arm more than the leg, and accompanied by slurred speech. MRI

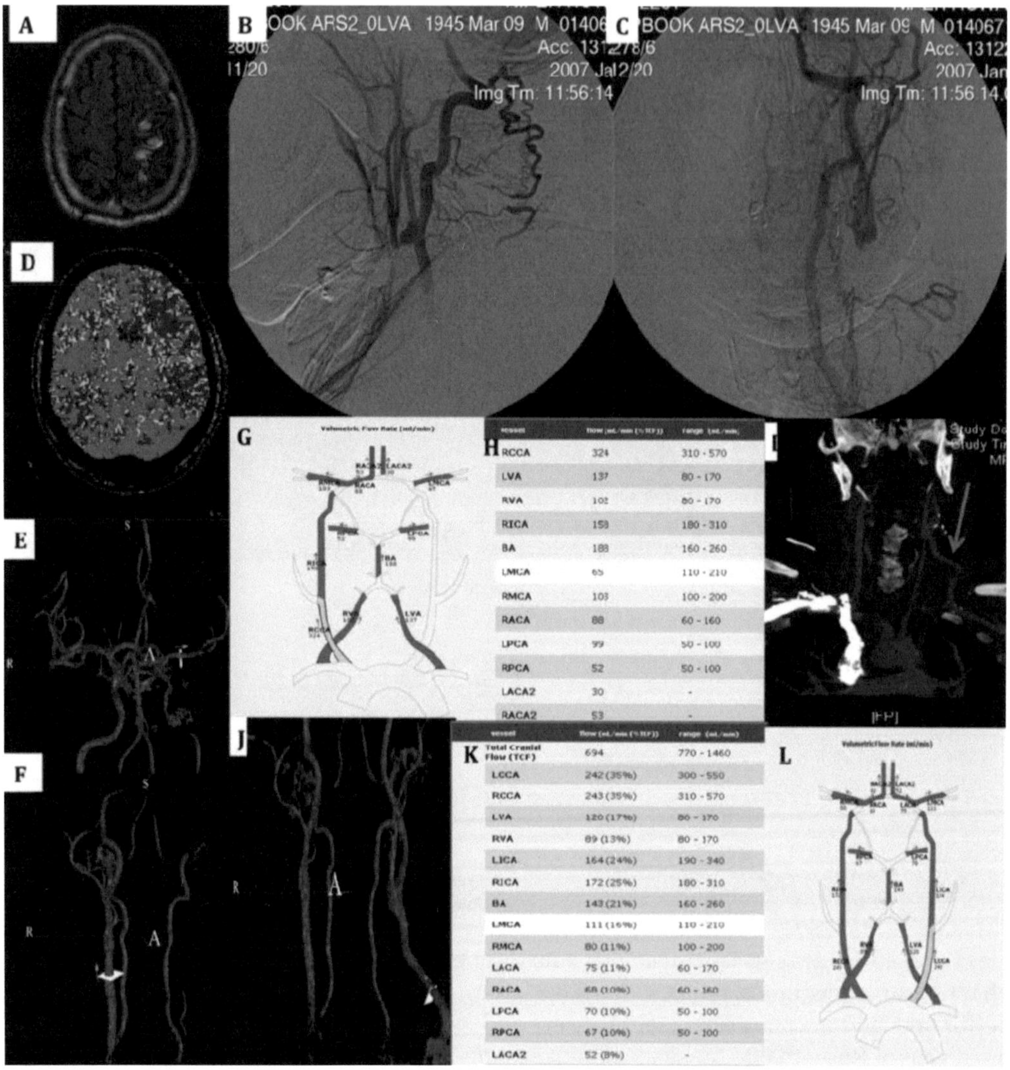

Fig. 2. Case 2 Images: A, Flair sequence MRI, axial section, shows a left hemisphere infarct. B, C, Lateral (B) and posterior-anterior (C) left vertebral angiogram shows reconstitution of the occluded left common carotid artery via cervicomuscular collaterals. D, CT perfusion scan after acetazolamide administration demonstrates decreased perfusion in the left MCA distribution. E, F, Pre-bypass NOVA 3D surface rendering shows absence of the left carotid artery in the cervical region and poor intracranial flow. G,H, Pre-bypass NOVA vessel map (G) and baseline table (H) show markedly abnormal flow in the left MCA and no flow in the left carotid artery. I, Coronal CTA after subclavian to carotid bulb bypass clearly demonstrates bypass patency. J, NOVA 3D rendering post-bypass shows the bypass with the cursor placed to measure flow. K, L, Post-bypass NOVA baseline table (K) and vessel map (L) demonstrate increased flow in the left MCA post-bypass, which is now in the normal range.

revealed an acute stroke in the left corona radiata consistent with a watershed infarction (Figure 2A). Further workup, including angiography, revealed an acute left common carotid occlusion with reconstitution of the carotid artery in the region of the carotid bulb via vertebral artery collaterals (Figure 2B,C). The patient was discharged home after near complete resolution of his hemiparesis and was referred for further evaluation because of the known carotid occlusion and daily recurrent episodes of visual loss in the left eye.

CT perfusion with acetazolamide challenge showed a persistent deficit in the left MCA territory (Figure 2D) and fundoscopy revealed optic neuropathy consistent with a chronic low-flow state. NOVA analysis showed decreased flow in the left MCA and no flow in the left common carotid (Figure 2E-H). The patient underwent a subclavian to common carotid bypass (Figure 2I). The patient's visual symptoms immediately resolved. Post-bypass NOVA showed good replacement flow in the bypass itself, good flow in the left ICA and normalization of flow in the left MCA (Figure 2J-L).

4.3 Case 3

This 52-year-old man with a history of hypertension, diabetes, hypercholesterolemia, coronary artery disease, and tobacco use had been placed on clopidogrel and aspirin after having multiple episodes of diplopia associated with hemisensory symptoms without infarct seen on MRI. After one such episode, imaging revealed bilateral occipital lobe, left cerebellar and right pontine acute infarctions (Figure 3A,B). Workup including CTA of the aortic arch, head and neck revealed multiple areas of irregular stenoses in the bilateral extracranial vertebral arteries. NOVA revealed diminished flow in both vertebral arteries with severely reduced flow in the left vertebral artery and basilar artery (Figure 3C).

Under general anesthesia, the patient underwent diagnostic angiography which confirmed the multiple irregular stenoses in the vertebral arteries and sluggish flow into the basilar artery and its distal branches (Figure 3D-E). The patient underwent balloon angioplasty of the left extracranial vertebral artery at the C1 level, the area felt to harbor the most severely stenotic and irregular segment. Balloon angioplasty was performed using the recently FDA-approved non-compliant Gateway balloon (Boston Scientific, Target) and was followed by placement of two telescoping recently FDA-approved WingSpan (Boston Scientific, Target) stents. This resulted in excellent angiographic dilatation with marked increased flow into the basilar artery and its tributaries (Figure 3F). This was confirmed by post-procedure NOVA (Figure 3G). The patient was discharged on clopidogrel and aspirin and did well with one readmission four months later for transient left facial numbness not associated with infarction. CTA performed at that time failed to reveal in-stent stenosis and MRI did not show an acute infarct and the patient was discharged home (Brisman, 2008).

4.4 Case 4

This 69 year old gentleman has a history of hypertension, hyperlipidemia and diabetes and three months prior to the current admission had an episode of vertigo and was found to have a right cerebellar and very small left cerebellar acute infarction (Fig. 4A). He made a good recovery and was discharged on clopidogrel. He was readmitted with episodes of diplopia and feeling unbalanced while walking. MRI showed bilateral cerebellar and occipital lobe small acute infarctions. CTA revealed a very focal area of vertebral artery

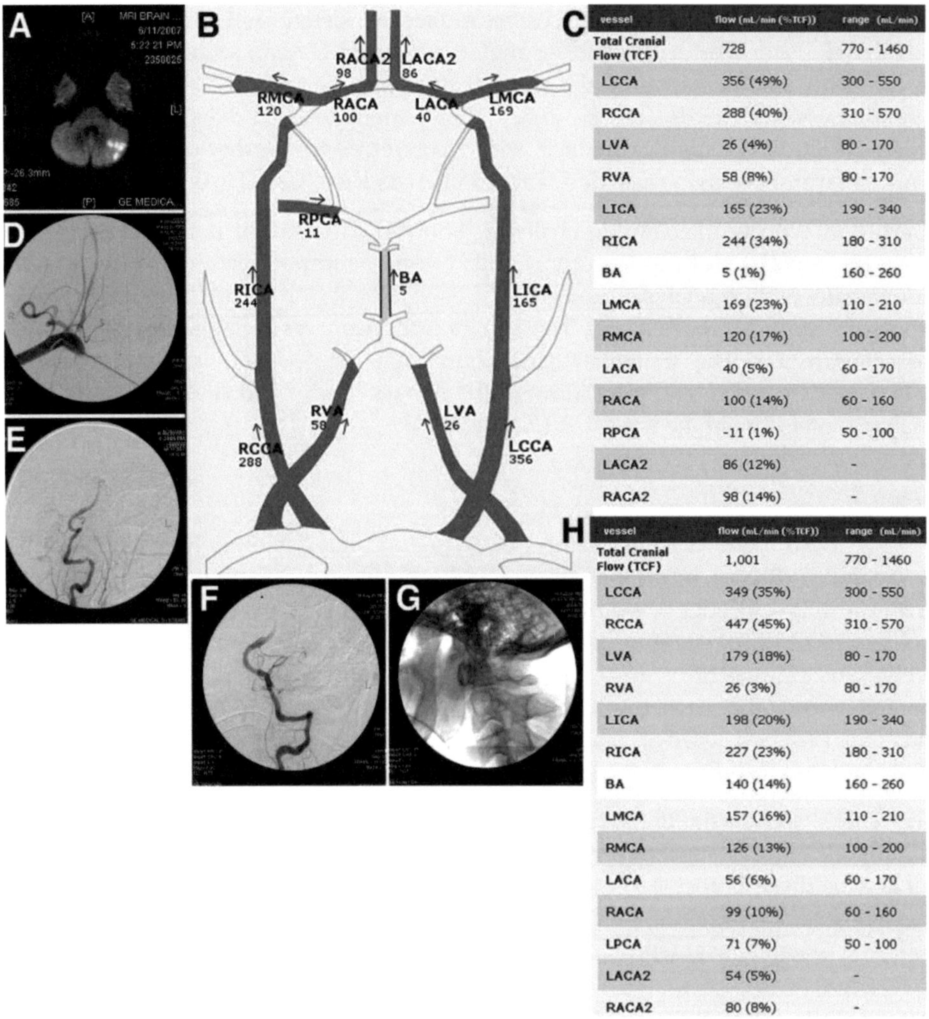

vessel	flow (mL/min (%TCF))	range (mL/min)
Total Cranial Flow (TCF)	728	770 - 1460
LCCA	356 (49%)	300 - 550
RCCA	288 (40%)	310 - 570
LVA	26 (4%)	80 - 170
RVA	58 (8%)	80 - 170
LICA	165 (23%)	190 - 340
RICA	244 (34%)	180 - 310
BA	5 (1%)	160 - 260
LMCA	169 (23%)	110 - 210
RMCA	120 (17%)	100 - 200
LACA	40 (5%)	60 - 170
RACA	100 (14%)	60 - 160
RPCA	-11 (1%)	50 - 100
LACA2	86 (12%)	-
RACA2	98 (14%)	-

vessel	flow (mL/min (%TCF))	range (mL/min)
Total Cranial Flow (TCF)	1,001	770 - 1460
LCCA	349 (35%)	300 - 550
RCCA	447 (45%)	310 - 570
LVA	179 (18%)	80 - 170
RVA	26 (3%)	80 - 170
LICA	198 (20%)	190 - 340
RICA	227 (23%)	180 - 310
BA	140 (14%)	160 - 260
LMCA	157 (16%)	110 - 210
RMCA	126 (13%)	100 - 200
LACA	56 (6%)	60 - 170
RACA	99 (10%)	60 - 160
LPCA	71 (7%)	50 - 100
LACA2	54 (5%)	-
RACA2	80 (8%)	-

Fig. 3. Case 3 Images: A: Diffusion-weighted brain MRI showing acute left cerebellar hemisphere infarction. B: QMRA (NOVA) flow map showing markedly diminished flow in both vertebral arteries (26 and 58 cc/min) and in the basilar (5 cc/min). R = right; L = left; MCA = middle cerebral artery; ACA = anterior cerebral artery; CCA = common carotid artery; ICA = internal carotid artery; BA = basilar artery and VA = vertebral artery. Directionality of blood flow is also given (arrows). C: QMRA (NOVA) flow table giving the values seen in the flow map with the "range" column representing expected normal values. D: Right subclavian artery angiogram, postero-anterior view, demonstrates severe right vertebral origin stenosis. E: Magnified oblique view of the left vertebral artery angiogram demonstrating stenotic irregular plaque in the high cervical vertebral artery. F: Successful angiographic reconstruction post-stent placement is seen on this left vertebral artery angiogram, oblique view. G: Cervical spine lateral x-ray demonstrates the two telescoping WingSpan stents placed at the C1 level of the vertebral artery. H: QMRA (NOVA) flow table demonstrating the marked increase in the left vertebral artery flow after stenting with resultant increase in basilar flow.

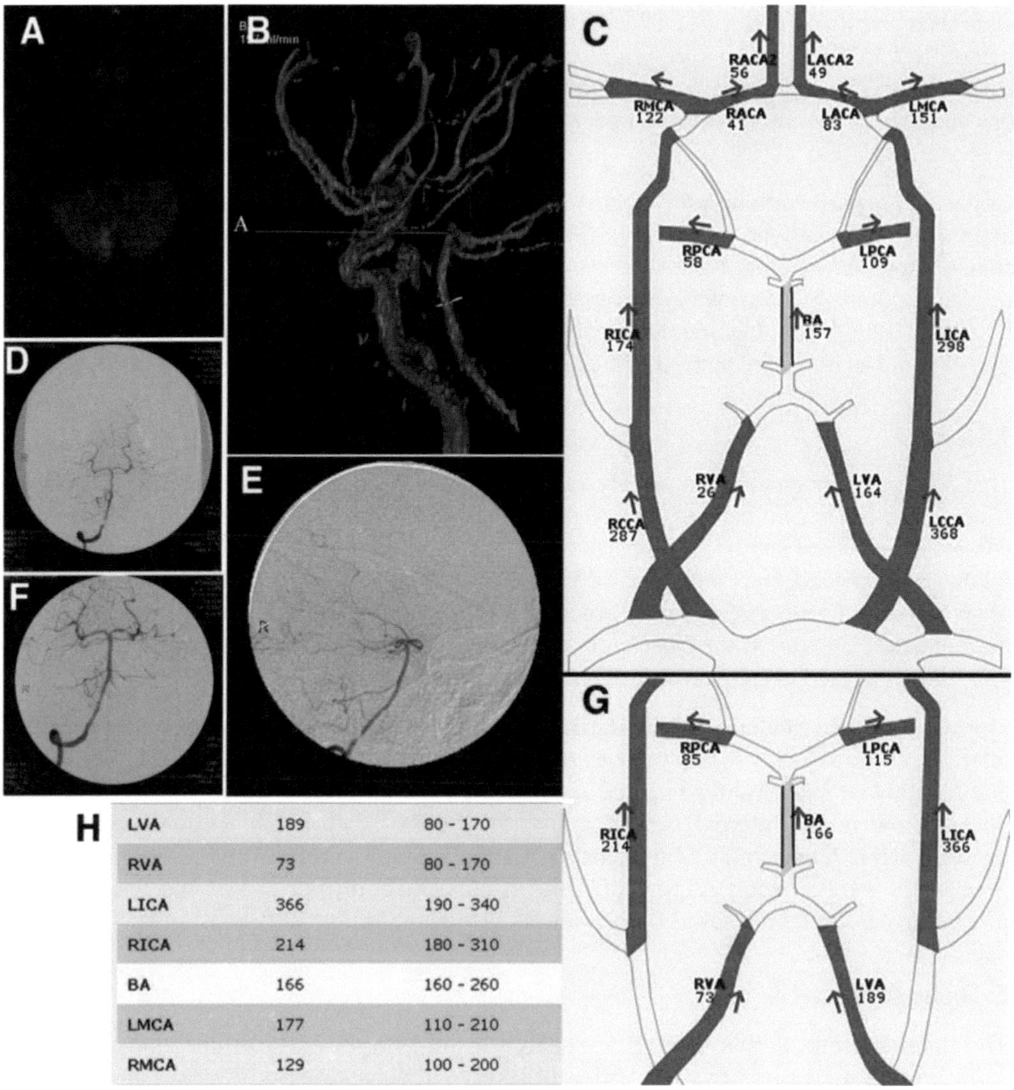

LVA	189	80 - 170
RVA	73	80 - 170
LICA	366	190 - 340
RICA	214	180 - 310
BA	166	160 - 260
LMCA	177	110 - 210
RMCA	129	100 - 200

Fig. 4. Case 4 Images: A: Diffusion-weighted brain MRI showing acute right cerebellar medial hemispheric infarction. B: NOVA MRA shows the region on the basilar artery (yellow line) where the flow was measured. Flow is normal (157 ml/min). C: QMRA (NOVA) flow map shows very low flow in the right vertebral artery (26 ml/min) compared with the non-stenotic left vertebral artery (164 ml/min). Again, normal flow in the basilar artery is seen. Abbreviations as defined in figure 2. D: Right vertebral artery postero-anterior angiogram demonstrates severe right vertebral stenosis proximal to its entrance intracranially. E: Right vertebral artery angiogram, lateral view, again demonstrates the stenotic lesion. F: Right vertebral artery angiogram, magnified lateral view, shows good angiographic result post-angioplasty and stent placement. G: QMRA (NOVA) flow map shows increased flow in the right vertebral artery post-stenting. H: QMRA (NOVA) flow table demonstrates that the flow in the right vertebral artery post-stenting approaches the expected normal values.

stenosis a small distance prior to its entrance into the foramen magnum. QMRA showed markedly diminished flow in the right vertebral artery compared with the left with normal basilar flow (Fig. 4B,C). The patient was taken for diagnostic angiography which confirmed one single very severe stenosis just proximal to the entrance of the vertebral artery into the posterior fossa (Fig. 4D,E).

Under full heparinization, a 6 French Envoy was navigated into the right vertebral artery and the Gateway balloon measuring 3.5mm X 15mm was used to perform angioplasty of the stenotic segment. Using the same 0.14 microguidewire for support, a WingSpan stent measuring 3mm X 15mm was deployed across the stenosis with good angiographic result (Fig. 4F). The QMRA documented increased flow in the right vertebral artery (Fig. 4G,H). The patient has remained symptom-free at the five-month follow-up (Brisman, 2008).

4.5 Case 5

This 36-year-old woman with history of migraine headaches was evaluated by a vascular surgeon for MRA findings suggestive of fibromuscular dysplasia (FMD). She was treated conservatively until she had two episodes of left hand incoordination over several months followed by several more episodes of left hand numbness and tingling. The attacks were often associated with anxiety and sometimes headaches and the diagnoses of complicated migraine and seizures were entertained. Her EEG did not suggest seizure activity and the episodes continued despite anticonvulsants.

Her MRA showed moderate right internal carotid stenosis over a long segment and mild left internal carotid stenosis with an associated kinking and small pseudoaneurysm (Figure 5A). NOVA showed significantly reduced flow in the internal carotid artery on the right with normal flow in the internal carotid artery on the left (Figure 4B). Formal angiography confirmed this (Figure 5C). She underwent right internal carotid artery angioplasty with good angiographic result (Figure 5D) and has not had further symptoms. NOVA post-procedure confirmed increased flow in the RICA (Figure 5E,F).

5. Discussion

The main finding of this chapter's research is that the NOVA commercially available software was used in a variety of different cerebrovascular disease processes and found to accurately represent the diagnosed pathophysiology and to reflect the expected changes of a therapeutic intervention. Excessive unexplained values outside of the company's quoted normal ranges render interpretation in a given study difficult and limit its utility at present. Since this study was completed, the company has issued more specific and hopefully more accurate normal control values based on their research suggesting alteration of expected normal values in different age populations. This study expands on a recently published study involving a subset of the current cohort in which arterial waveform analysis was shown to correlate with a neurovascular intervention (Brisman et al., 2011) We look forward to further evaluation of this technology using these new baselines. Although there are currently several good imaging modalities with which to study the cervico-cerebral vasculature (including ultrasound, CTA, MRA), these tests yield static images at one point in time. Catheter-based angiography can offer additional information about pace of blood flow and collateralization, but because of the invasiveness of the procedure there continues

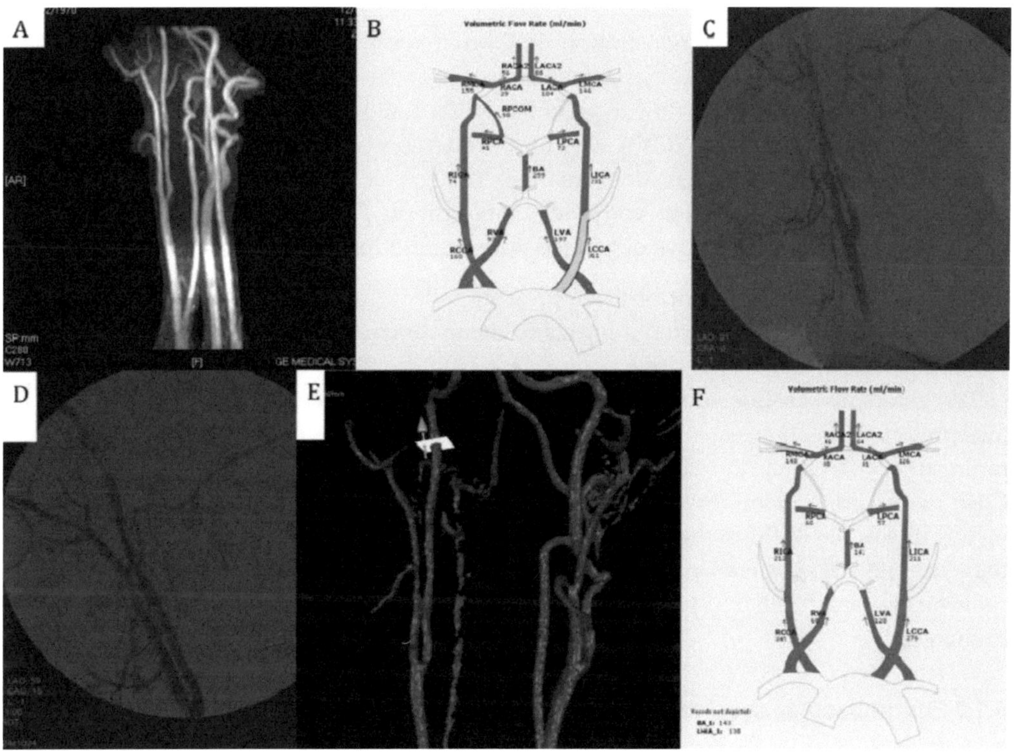

Fig. 5. Case 5 Images: A, MRA of the cervical vasculature demonstrates a right internal carotid long segment narrowing with a focal area of severe stenosis as well as a left internal carotid artery kink with an associated aneurysm in this patient with presumed FMD. B, Pre-angioplasty NOVA vessel map documents marked decrease in flow in the right internal carotid artery. C, Right common carotid angiogram, oblique view, pre-angioplasty (C) and post-angioplasty (D) shows excellent revascularization. E, NOVA 3D surface rendering of the cervical vasculature post-angioplasty appears strikingly similar to the angiogram in D. F, NOVA vessel map post-angioplasty documents marked increase in flow in the right internal carotid artery.

to be a search for less invasive modalities that can give similar or better information. Techniques such as SPECT, Xenon-CT, TCD, PET, CT Perfusion, and MR Perfusion offer an assessment of cerebrovascular physiology, but do not give quantitative information of blood flow in specific vessels. NOVA represents the only commercially available method to quantify cervico-cerebral blood flow utilizing standard MRI platforms.

5.1 NOVA in specific disease entities

5.1.1 Radiosurgery of brain AVMs

This represents the first demonstration of QMRA for brain AVMs as well as the first demonstration of QMRA changes after radiosurgery in brain AVMs. Prior attempts to noninvasively measure blood flow in vascular malformations have been restricted to the use of ultrasound. In one study NOVA was used to demonstrate the efficacy of endovascular embolization of Vein of Galen Malformations (Langer et al., 2006b). In the two reported cases NOVA performed before and after embolization documented marked decrease in blood flow in draining veins that correlated with angiographic findings.

In the current report, two out of three patients with brain AVMs demonstrated marked increased flow in the main arterial inputs to the malformation with asymmetric increased blood flow in the transverse sinus system receiving the AVM venous drainage. Currently NOVA offers no baseline values for blood flow in the dural venous sinuses. Therefore, the interpretation of changes in blood flow in the venous sinus system six months after radiosurgery is based on relative and not absolute values and is of unclear significance. Clear decreases in blood flow in all three cases in the draining sinuses, more pronounced on the side of the AVM in the two non-midline lesions, was used to counsel these patients that despite no change in the AVM appearance on routine brain MRI, that the radiosurgery may be having an effect as evidenced by decreased blood flow in the venous drainage.

5.1.2 Fibromuscular dysplasia and carotid stenosis

This represents the first study documenting NOVA flow measurements in two patients with FMD and carotid stenosis (CS) and the first to demonstrate changes in NOVA after carotid angioplasty in one affected patient. Ghogawala et al. (2008) demonstrated increased flow following carotid endarterectomy in a patient with carotid stenosis using NOVA. They also showed that diminished blood flow from carotid stenosis correlated with improved cognitive outcomes after revascularization and suggested that quantification of blood flow before and after revascularization using NOVA may be an important way to study the effects of the intervention (Brisman, 2008). While CS secondary to atherosclerotic disease has been well studied, carotid steno-occlusive disease in patients with fibromuscular dysplasia is a less familiar entity. Whereas CS from atherosclerosis is felt to cause symptoms from thrombo-embolism, this is not the case with FMD, where decreased flow may play more of a role. This probably reflects the different histologic pathology between the two diseases. As a result, treatment options for patients with CS and FMD have been more controversial, reflecting our lack of understanding of the natural history risks as well as the treatment risk of either open or endovascular options.

Various open surgical treatments have been used historically for CS in patients with FMD, ranging from surgical exposure and angioplasty under direct vision to excision of the diseased segment and patching. Currently, endovascular angioplasty is the most popular treatment for symptomatic CS in FMD patients and its success parallels that in the renal vasculature of such patients. FMD patients with asymptomatic CS represent a group in which no clear recommendations exist. In cases of moderate to severe stenosis, NOVA may provide the best way to follow such patients. At what point to intervene based on changes in NOVA flow remains an unanswered question. Based on our two cases, NOVA documented clearly decreased flow with marked increase after angioplasty in the one patient treated.

5.1.3 Vasospasm after SAH

Cerebral vasospasm after aneurysmal subarachnoid hemorrhage remains the most significant source of morbidity and mortality in these patients, with an estimated one sixth of all patients developing permanent disability. While the exact etiology and pathophysiology of the process is unknown, screening and detection using transcranial dopplers, computed tomographic angiography and catheter angiography are well described and important as treatment options that may avert stroke are available.

By quantifying blood flow in spastic vessels, NOVA may be a better method with which to detect and follow vasospasm as well as assess instituted therapies. Transcranial doppler ultrasonography and CTA yield anatomic information only and are therefore poor predictors of who will develop symptomatic vasospasm. Angiography is somewhat invasive, is impractical to perform multiple times during the vasospasm period and also generates mostly anatomic information.

NOVA appeared to correlate with CTA and angiography in the one patient studied. This is the first demonstration of vasospasm using NOVA. A modified abridged version of the NOVA was performed on this patient in which only three vessels were studied: the basilar artery and both MCA arteries. The intent was to reduce the time required for the test (to under 10 minutes) such that it would be practical for critically ill patients such as those who have suffered subarachnoid hemorrhage and may have vasospasm. Additionally it made sense to study only these vessels as it is only in these vessels that balloon angioplasty is generally performed in cases of medically refractory vasospasm. Further studies evaluating larger numbers of patients and looking at additional vessels, particularly the anterior cerebral and supraclinoid carotid arteries, might also be important.

5.1.4 Vascular bypass for ischemia

NOVA was used to study two patients who underwent extracranial-intracranial bypass as part of a cerebrovascular augmentation procedure in the setting of unilateral carotid occlusion, ipsilateral symptoms and documented poor cerebrovascular reserve. The use of NOVA to study the integrity and potential utility of bypass for occlusive ischemic disease has been previously studied by Amin-Hanjani et al. when they reviewed 101 bypasses in which they performed NOVA before and after. They showed that NOVA was a good way to document the integrity of the graft and to follow it over time (Amin-Hanjani et al., 2007).

In our patient with a subclavian-carotid bypass, NOVA readily measured flow in the graft and documented increased intracranial flow compared to the patient's presurgical state. In the patient with the STA-MCA bypass, despite patency on angiographic imaging, NOVA could not measure flow in the graft, suggesting that the flow was too low to be detected or technical error of the NOVA. NOVA requires a certain size vessel to obtain measurements. As the graft matures, future NOVA studies may be able to detect and measure flow.

5.1.5 Atherosclerotic disease and endovascular revascularization

NOVA was used in four patients with vertebrobasilar ischemia, two from severe basilar artery stenosis and two from extradural vertebral stenosis. In three out of four patients, the authors considered NOVA to be CD. One of the patients with vertebral disease had a solitary focus and the other had multiple lesions. In the two patients with basilar stenosis and very low flow in the basilar artery (cases 3 and 4), results of NOVA were used to recommend balloon angioplasty and stent placement despite the patients not having failed maximal medical therapy. The justification for this was based on the results of one study that used NOVA flow in the basilar and posterior cerebral arteries to predict which patients with vertebrobasilar ischemia would benefit from posterior circulation revascularization as opposed to medical therapy (Amin-Hanjani et al., 2005). Both patients declined interventional treatment.

Cases 3 and 4 document the utilization of the new WingSpan stent and Gateway balloon system to treat two patients with medically refractory vertebrobasilar ischemia secondary to cervical vertebral artery stenosis. The self-expanding nitinol stent is designed for use after balloon angioplasty using a specially designed balloon and has not been previously described in the treatment of extracranial vertebral artery disease (Brisman, 2008).

This is the first description of the use of this novel stent for the treatment of the extracranial vertebral arteries as well as the first documentation of QMRA before and after WingSpan stenting of any vessel (Brisman, 2008).

Historically, extracranial vertebral artery disease had been treated with surgical bypass (Spetzler et al., 1987) but has since given way to endovascular approaches. This shift reflects the technical difficulty and unfamiliarity of most neurosurgeons with the former and the improved success and experience with the latter. Stenting and angioplasty has been well described for the extracranial vertebral arteries (Ko et al., 2004 & Malek et al., 1999) with some success with both balloon-mounted coronary stents and self-expanding stents designed for non-cerebral revascularization. Such stents can be difficult to navigate due to the tortuosity of the cervico-cerebral vasculature and associated with complication rates (4.8% major morbidity in one series) (Malek et al., 1999) that may relate to the difficulty with stent delivery, overly aggressive balloon angioplasty and/or excessive radial force during deployment or afterwards. Recurrent events post-stenting (persistent in 9.5% in one series) (Malek et al., 1999) and high rates of restenosis (10-43%) (Ko et al., 2004) suggest that current endovascular options may be improved upon. The WingSpan stent system and Gateway balloon were specifically designed to access and treat more fragile intracranial vessels. The seminal safety study of this stent used in 45 patients with medically refractory intracranial stenosis was recently published (Bose et al., 2007). Although not specifically designed for extracranial disease, the system was employed with technical ease and success in the two patients here described.

In addition to this technical success associated with very acceptable angiographic results, QMRA demonstrated expected increases in flow in the treated vertebral artery in both patients. That said, one patient did have an episode several months later of transient facial numbness that may have represented a posterior circulation transient ischemic attack. This patient, however, has multiple risk factors for vasculopathic disease and stenting was directed to the most stenotic and irregular region of the vertebral artery. If such episodes persist, consideration may be given to treatment of his additional vertebral stenoses. Another caveat of this system is the issue of in-stent restenosis, which has been well described for vertebral artery stents, and which was not addressed in this report. As the clinical follow-up is short and no catheter angiographic follow-up has been presented, the durability of the WingSpan stent in the extracranial vertebral arteries remains unknown. QMRA may prove useful to follow such patients post-stenting as decreased flows may herald restenosis.

Currently there are several very good imaging modalities with which to study the anatomy of the cervico-cerebral vasculature. These include ultrasound (carotid duplex and transcranial duplex), CTA, MRA and catheter angiography and range from non-invasive (duplex, MRA) to minimally invasive (CTA) to invasive with low risk (catheter angiography). Those studies that are minimally or non-invasive, however, yield static images, and despite tremendous advances in the ability to manipulate these images, the studies do not give more than a picture of the vascular anatomy at one point in time. Catheter angiography offers specific additional information about cervico-cerebral vascular pathology such as pace of blood flow and collateralization. Because of the invasiveness of the procedure, however, there has been a continued search for less invasive modalities that might offer similar or better information. Additional modalities have been developed, therefore, using a wide range of techniques, that attempt to give some assessment of cerebrovascular physiology. Such techniques include SPECT, Xenon-CT, TCD, PET, CT Perfusion, and MR Perfusion. None of these studies gives quantitative information of blood flow. NOVA is a software package that represents the only commercially available technique to quantify cervico-cerebral blood flow utilizing standard MRI platforms. It has been shown to effectively risk-stratify patients with vertebrobasilar ischemia based on distal flow in the basilar and posterior cerebral arteries (Amin-Hanjani et al., 2005).

In these two cases, vessel dilatation post-procedure was associated with an expected increase in flow values. Interestingly, in one of the two cases, basilar flow was normal, suggesting the lesion was not flow-limiting. Stent placement in that patient might have more efficacy as an intimal stabilizer against further thrombo-embolic events, whereas in the other patient flow-limitation and thrombo-embolism were both probably contributing to ischemia (Brisman, 2008).

5.2 Caveats to this study and limitations of NOVA

Some of the findings of this study are objective, such as the common occurrence of abnormal values that lacks a simple explanation. Our study surprisingly showed a 41% false positive rate, bringing into question the validity of the software. It is possible, however, that we did not appreciate that the abnormal flow in a given vessel was part of the pathologic process. Additionally, it is possible that the defined "normal values" from the company need adjustment. The more subjective part of this report involves the designation of HP, CD or NUD to a given NOVA test. This designation is multifactorial and incorporates our understanding of the disease process, the kinds of patients evaluated and referred for NOVA testing and threshold for intervention.

There are quite a few limitations of the NOVA technology, some of which likely are preventing its adoption into mainstream cerebrovascular care. The most prominent problem is the lack of properly defined baseline normal values, as mentioned above. The baseline values provided by the company are based on a large cohort of healthy volunteers. The company is currently studying another large group of volunteers in an effort to better define baseline values (personal communication). Particular clarification is needed with regard to defining the range of normal values and what, if any, adjustments should be made for certain patient-specific factors such as age (which has recently been addressed), cardiac dysfunction or dehydration, to name just a few. Is there a range of fluctuation in NOVA values that is acceptable for a given individual at different periods of the day or seasonally? Do NOVA results vary in relation to meals or with patients who are febrile, diabetics or smokers? All these questions will need to be answered in order to make the appropriate adjustments such that true pathologic states can be ascertained across a wide spectrum of patients. These caveats not withstanding, we do believe that the findings here of alteration in flow in an expected manner for those patients undergoing an intervention is significant but agree that further validation of the basic software is in order.

6. Conclusion

NOVA represents the only currently available method to non-invasively quantify blood flow in the human cervico-cerebral vasculature and will likely play a more prominent role in cerebrovascular care as research better defines expected values for different patient populations at baseline and in disease states. This study represents the largest clinical experience using NOVA in a routine cerebrovascular practice encompassing diverse pathologies. Analyses of NOVA in certain conditions, such as radiosurgery of brain AVMs, carotid stenosis from fibromuscular dysplasia, and vasospasm after aneurysmal subarachnoid hemorrhage have not been previously described. We found NOVA to accurately reflect expected blood flow changes before and after a neurovascular intervention in all cases. Further research into this new technology that better defines expected normal and disease state values will likely result in increased incorporation into mainstream cerebrovascular practice.

7. References

Amin-Hanjani S, Du X, Zhao M, Walsh K, Malisch TW, & Charbel FT. (2005). Use of quantitative magnetic resonance angiography to stratify stroke risk in symptomatic vertebrobasilar disease. *Stroke*, 36:1140-1145.

Amin-Hanjani S, Shin JH, Zhao M, Du X, & Charbel FT. (2007). Evaluation of extracranial-intracranial bypass using quantitative magnetic resonance angiography. *J Neurosurg,* 106:291-298.

Bauer AM, Amin-Hanjani S, Alaraj A, & Charbel FT. (2008). Quantitative magnetic resonance angiography in the evaluation of the subclavian steal syndrome: Report of 5 patients. *J Neuroimaging.*

Bose A, Hartmann M, Henkes H, Liu HM, Teng MH, Szikora I, et al. (2007). A novel, self-expanding, nitinol stent in medically refractory intracranial atherosclerotic stenoses: The WingSpan Study. *Stroke,* 38:1531-7.

Brisman JL. (2008). Wingspan stenting of symptomatic extracranial vertebral artery stenosis and perioperative evaluation using quantitative magnetic resonance angiography: report of two cases. *Neurosurg Focus,* 24:E14.

Brisman JL, Pile-Spellman J, & Konstas AA. (2011). Clinical utility of quantitative magnetic resonance angiography in the assessment of the underlying pathophysiology in a variety of cerebrovascular disorders. *European Journal of Radiology,* in press/e-published.

Charbel FT, Zhao M, Amin-Hanjani S, Hoffman W, Du X, & Clark ME. (2004). A patient-specific computer model to predict outcomes of the balloon occlusion test. *J Neurosurg,* 101:977-988.

Ghogawala Z, Westerveld M, & Amin-Hanjani S. (2008). Cognitive outcomes after carotid revascularization: the role of cerebral emboli and hypoperfusion. *Neurosurgery,* 62:385-395.

Ko YG, Park S, Kim JY, Min PK, Choi EY, Jung JH, et al. (2004). Percutaneous interventional treatment of extracranial vertebral artery stenosis with coronary stents. *Yonsei Med J,* 45(4):629-634.

Langer DJ, Lefton DR, Ostergren L, Brockington CD, Song J, Niimi Y, Bhargava P, & Berenstein A. (2006 (a.)). Hemispheric revascularization in the setting of carotid occlusion and subclavian steal: a diagnostic and management role for quantitative magnetic resonance angiography? *Neurosurgery,* 58:528-533.

Langer DJ, Song JK, Niimi Y, Chwajol M, Lefton DR, Brisman JL, Molofsky W, Kupersmith MJ, & Berenstein A. (2006 (b.)). Transarterial embolization of vein of Galen malformations: the use of magnetic resonance imaging noninvasive optimal vessel analysis to quantify shunt reduction. Report of two cases. *J Neurosurg,* 104:41-45.

Malek AM, Higashida RT, Phatouros CC, Lempert TE, Meyers PM, Gress DR, et al. (1999). Treatment of posterior circulation ischemia with extracranial percutaneous balloon angioplasty and stent placement. *Stroke,* 10:2073-85.

Prabhakaran S, Warrior L, Wells KR, Jhaveri MD, Chen M, & Lopes DK. (2009). The utility of quantitative magnetic resonance angiography in the assessment of intracranial in-stent stenosis. *Stroke.*

Ruland S, Ahmed A, Thomas K, Zhao M, Amin-Hanjani S, Du X, & Charbel FT. (2008). Leptomeningeal collateral volume flow assessed by quantitative magnetic resonance angiography in large-vessel cerebrovascular disease. *J Neuroimaging.*

Spetzler RF, Hadley MN, Martin NA, Hopkins LN, Carter LP, & Budny J. (1987). Vertebrobasilar insufficiency. Part 1: Microsurgical treatment of extracranial vertebrobasilar disease. *J Neurosurg*, 66(5):648-61.

Zhao M, Charbel FT, Alperin N, Loth F, & Clark ME. (2000). Improved phase-contrast flow quantification by three-dimensional vessel localization. *Magn Reson Imaging*, 18:697-706.

Part 3

MRA of the Aorta and Peripheral Arterial Tree

6

Magnetic Resonance Angiography of Aortic Diseases in Children

Shobhit Madan, Soma Mandal and Sameh S. Tadros
Division of Pediatric Radiology
Department of Radiology
Children's Hospital of Pittsburgh of UPMC
University of Pittsburgh School of Medicine
Pittsburgh, PA
USA

1. Introduction

Magnetic resonance angiography (MRA), a non-invasive, radiation-free imaging technique dependent on the body's natural magnetic properties in blood vessels, investigates abnormalities within the aorta. MRA is generally divided into Gadolinium (Gd) based contrast enhanced MRA (CE-MRA) and non-contrast enhanced MRA (NCE-MRA), used for both qualitative and quantitative assessment of the aorta. These sequences can be exemplified with a variety of aortic abnormalities including aortic dissection, coarctation of the aorta, genetic disorders with aortic pathologies (e.g., Marfan's syndrome, Loeys-Dietz syndrome), ascending and descending aortic aneurysms, Takayasu Arteritis, and various anomalies concerning the aortic arch as well as the aortic valve. While MRA can be applied to nearly any vessel in the body, the primary objective of this chapter is to focus on the role of MRA in the accurate quantitative and qualitative assessment of congenital and acquired aortic diseases. In many hospitals, a significant number of patients who are referred to MRA imaging is comprised of patients with aortic diseases, especially coarctation of aorta [Taylor, 2008]. The diagnostic utility of MRA is illustrated by a variety of pediatric aortic abnormalities.

2. Magnetic resonance angiography sequences

Examination of the aorta can be classified under purely qualitative imaging and both qualitative and quantitative imaging.

2.1 Qualitative aortic angiography

The first basic sequence employed is the non-electrocardiographic (ECG) gated steady-state free precision (SSFP) localizers in the coronal, axial and sagittal planes to visualize the entire chest and upper abdomen, providing a basic overview of cardiac and visceral situs and cardiovascular anatomy (Figure 1A-C). The localizers serve as the starting point for further disease-specific multiplanar image acquisition of the aorta for morphological, functional, and hemodynamic evaluation. Black-blood imaging, where the flowing blood appears dark and general aortic anatomy can be assessed, is exclusively used for qualitative analysis of the aortic morphology in multiple planes (Figure 1D-F). Black blood imaging includes a T1-weighted spin echo sequence (which allows for rapid aortic morphological assessment at low spatial resolution) followed by a double inversion recovery spin echo sequence (which allows for high spatial resolution and improved blood-myocardium contrast) in order to characterize cardiovascular tissue and assess airway obstruction.

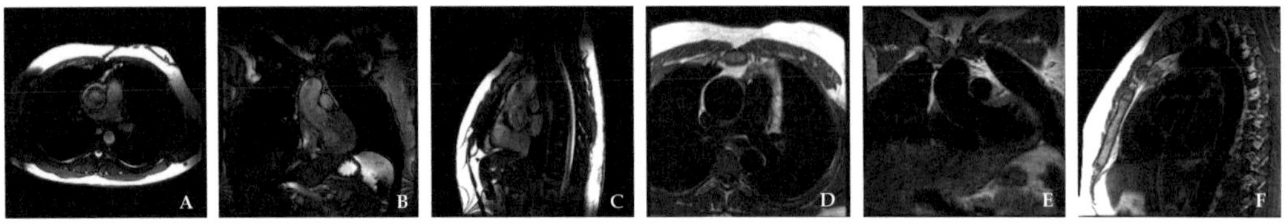

Fig. 1. SSFP localizer images demonstrating the aorta in axial (A), coronal (B), and sagittal (C) planes; Black-blood images demonstrating the aorta in axial (D), coronal (E), and sagittal (F) planes.

2.2 Quantitative & qualitative aortic angiography

In assessing the aorta both qualitatively and quantitatively, the cardiac imager may have two intentions in the quantitative measurement of vessels. On one hand, the imager can measure hemodynamic parameters such as blood flow, which would be accomplished more thoroughly by sequences which are concerned with functional assessment. On the other hand, more static measurements, such as assessing aortic root dilatation, would be accomplished more readily with sequences dedicated to morphological assessment. The following qualitative and quantitative sequences are discussed below.

Functional Assessment

A popular sequence used for functional assessment is the SSFP cine white blood imaging sequence, which provides superior quantitative imaging of the aorta and its branch vessels [Finn et al., 2006] without the use of contrast agents with high temporal resolution in multiple planes (Figure 2).

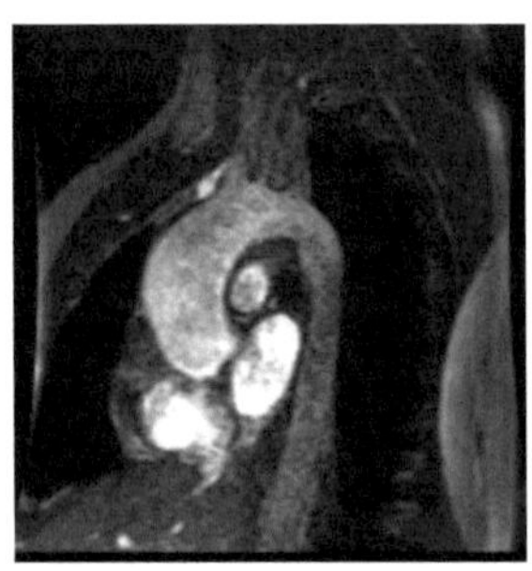

Fig. 2. SSFP cine image demonstrating aorta in a sagittal plane.

SSFP imaging is very useful in qualitative assessment of aortic valve for regurgitation and stenosis. This technique requires breath-hold which is necessary to improve image quality by avoiding motion artifacts. Post processing of SSFP images includes assessment of 3D computational fluid dynamics (CFD). CFD simulation of hemodynamics in aortic arch models allows for quantification of high resolution internal flow fields (e.g. velocity, pressure) as well as useful flow derived parameter such as time resolved wall shear stress, energy dissipation and power loss (Figure 3). Flow derived parameters have application in surgical planning and post-operative assessment of hemodynamic efficiency in surgical anastomosis or venous flow confluences [Lara et al., 2011]. CFD is a powerful tool for simulation of altered hemodynamics in pathological anatomies and may be used to assess aortic arch abnormalities, severity of coarctation (via assessment of pressure gradients, collateral flow, and velocity across the coarctation), and flow in arch anomalies (e.g. hypoplastic arch).

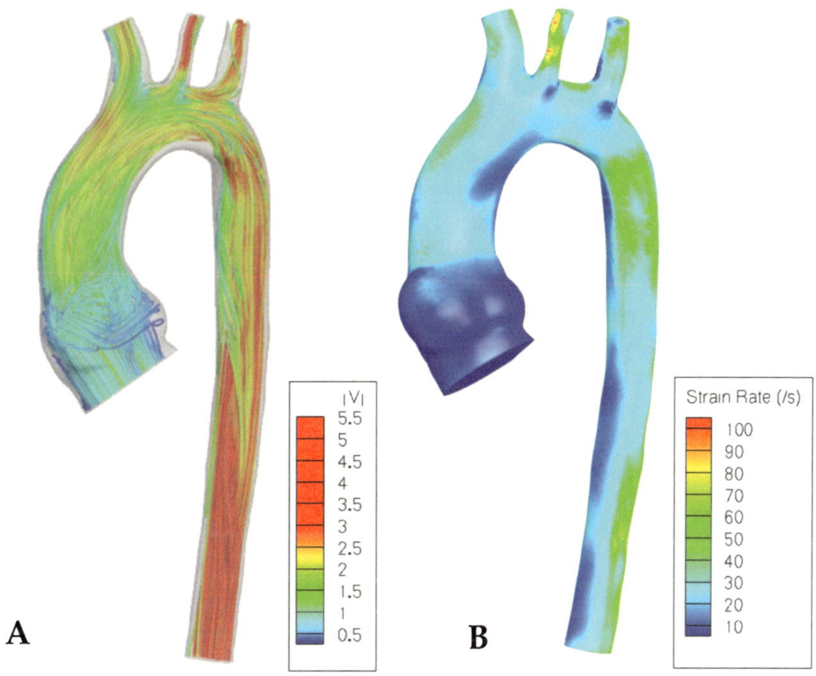

Fig. 3. Cine MRI based surface model reconstructions of a normal neonatal arch [Pekkan et al. 2008] were used to conduct 3D CFD and assess vascular flow. (A) Streamlines colored by inlet normalized velocity magnitude, | V |, for a mean steady aortic root velocity of 0.33 m/s; B) Wall shear strain rate, with an observed stain rate is within normal ranges for neonatal flow.

Another functional imaging sequence is velocity-encoded cine phase contrast imaging (Figure 4). Phase contrast imaging is a method of obtaining quantitative information on blood flow, in addition to providing anatomic imaging of vessels. Its mechanics depend on magnetic moments, or spins, which ultimately shift in their phase of rotation, allowing for a voxel specific velocity to be calculated and an image to be formed [Lotz et al., 2002; Sena 2008]. Quantification of flow at multiple levels of the aorta can be performed with and without breath holding using this technique. Determination of collateral flow, velocity, and pressure gradient across the coarctation in patients with coarctation of aorta can be preformed using this MR technique.

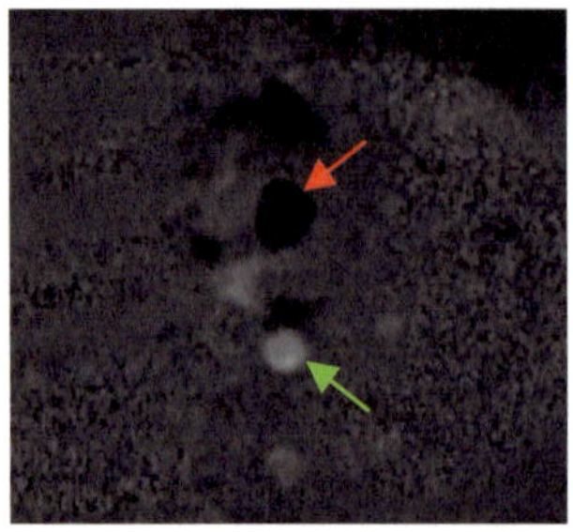

Fig. 4. Phase contrast image of the aorta demonstrating flow in the ascending aorta (red arrow) and descending aorta (green arrow) which is quantifiable as demonstrated in Figure. 14D later in the chapter.

Morphological Assessment

Traditional imaging of MRA includes both Gd-based CE-MRA as well as NCE-MRA using 3D SSFP, both of which serve as the source images for further post-processing which allows for static measurements and the creation of 3D models.

Gd-based CE-MRA has certain technical advantages over non-contrast enhanced MRA including superior visualization of vasculature, shorter acquisition times, and being less prone to alteration by motion artifacts [Hartung et al., 2011]. CE-MRA is considered the most quick and efficient way of illustrating the entire thoracic vasculature (Figure 5A); high resolution spatial techniques within this sequence are especially beneficial in imaging the small vasculature of newborns with specific aortic malformations like truncus arteriosus [Sena et al., 2008]. The ability to reconstruct maximum intensified projection (MIP) images (Figure 5B), volume rendered (VR) images (Figure 5C), and curved planar reformatted images allows for accurate measurements of vascular dimensions and aortic anatomy in patients with congenital and acquired aortic diseases. Limitations of CE-MRA techniques include the presence of motion artifacts in patients unable to breath-hold and patients with history of contrast agent allergies. A long-term complication of Nephrogenic Systemic Fibrosis in patients with poor renal function is another limitation of CE-MRA. Patients with metabolic syndromes, diabetes, and renal disease are especially at high risk and complications in these patients have spurred research with more diluted doses of contrast agents [Perazella et al., 2009].

With recent technical advancements in aortic imaging, NCE-MRA using 3D SSFP with and without breath hold imaging aids in the qualitative and quantitative assessment of the aorta with excellent spatial resolution without the need for Gd based contrast agents (Figure 5D). This advanced cardiovascular MRA sequence is especially useful in patients with a contraindication to contrast agents or who are unable to hold their breath. Measurements of the aorta and its branch vessels along with 3D and MIP image reconstructions in multiple planes are also possible with high accuracy using this sequence. A type of NCE-MRA, which will not be discussed in this chapter, is time of flight (TOF) MRA, which is based off of inflow effects, is a technique which is limited by longer acquisition time and a higher incidence of artifacts.

Additionally, late gadolinium enhancement (LGE) is a method by which regions of inflammation and fibrosis in the wall of aorta and its branch vessels can be identified. LGE,

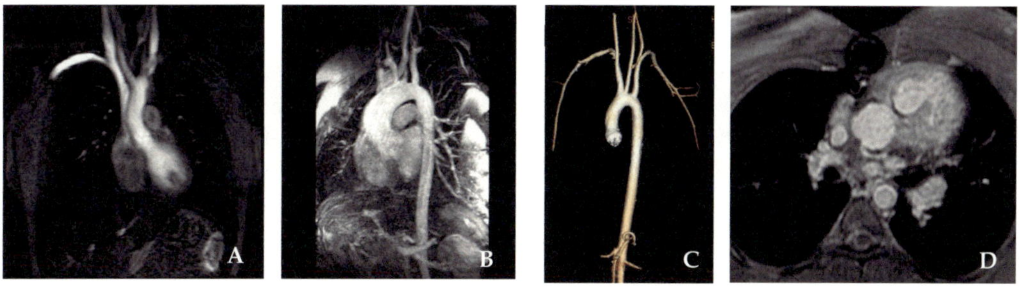

Fig. 5. CE-MRA coronal image (A), MIP sagittal reconstruction of CE-MRA (B), VR sagittal reconstruction of CE-MRA (C), and axial NCE-MRA image using 3D SSFP (D) of the aorta. MIP and VR reconstructions are extremely useful for a qualitative overview of the vascular morphology for preoperative assessment.

a sequence that visualizes fibrotic or infarcted heart tissue, derives its name from the fact that there is a delay in the washout of gadolinium-based contrast because fibrotic regions are filled with collagen. It was first demonstrated in the late 1980s with animal models demonstrating enhancement of myocardial infarcts [van Dijkman et al., 1989]. In recent decades, LGE has been shown to be particularly useful in pediatric diseases [Prakash et al., 2003]. However, the exact mechanism of contrast agent localization in infarcted tissue is a debated topic [Finn et al., 2006].

As mentioned, MRA can be utilized to image nearly any vessel in the body. The following table is a concise summary of current MRA techniques used for imaging of various vessels in the body, with sequences like black blood, phase contrast, SSFP, and ECG-gated fast spin echo (which is a variation of SSFP which we have not discussed in the chapter due to its irregular and sparse use), which are specifically used for aortic imaging [Morita et al., 2011].

Advantages, Limitations, and Clinical Applications of Unenhanced MR Angiographic Techniques

Technique	Advantages	Limitations	Clinical Applications
TOF	Simple and robust	Long imaging time; direction dependent; signal loss in in-plane, turbulent, or complex flow; susceptible to field heterogeneities	Cerebral arteries (3D), peripheral vessels (2D), head and neck arteries (2D)
Phase-contrast	Suppressed background signals, direction independent	Long imaging time (3D), signal loss in turbulent flow, sensitive to motion, parameter dependent	Cerebral veins (3D), hemodynamic evaluation
ECG-gated FSE	Relatively short imaging time, sensitive to slow flow, less susceptible to field heterogeneities	Complex imaging, direction dependent, sensitive to motion	Peripheral arteries, aorta
SSFP	Short imaging time, high signal-to-noise ratio, relatively flow independent	High background signals, susceptible to field heterogeneities	Renal arteries, aorta, coronary arteries
ASL with SSFP	High signal-to-noise ratio, suppressed background signals	Relatively complex imaging, signal loss in fast or complex flow, susceptible to field heterogeneities	Renal arteries, various visceral vessels
Black blood	Less sensitive to complex flow	Long imaging time, unsuitable for angiography	Vessel wall imaging, carotid arteries, aorta

Note.—ASL = arterial spin labeling, ECG = electrocardiograph, FSE = fast spin echo, SSFP = steady-state free precession, 3D = three-dimensional, 2D = two-dimensional.

3. Diseases of the aorta

Various diseases of the aorta, primarily highlighted in the pediatric population due to the large volume of pediatric cases in our institution as well as the congenital presentation of most of the diseases, are illustrated with the sequences discussed above. In general, almost all aortic diseases will be imaged via black-blood, CE-MRA, SSFP, phase contrast, and post-processed to MIP and VR images as necessary for a comprehensive assessment available for the cardiac imager, cardiologist, or the surgeon.

3.1 Coarctation of aorta

Coarctation of aorta, a congenital condition characterized by aortic narrowing, is subtyped based on the location of the narrowing relative to the ductus arteriosus. The use of MRA in determining the severity of stenosis within aortic coarctation is well documented [Nielsen et al., 2005; Muzzarelli et al., 2011; Secchi et al., 2009]. Coarctation of aorta requires comprehensive qualitative and quantitative evaluation for the assessment of severity of coarctation (e.g. velocity measurements at the level of coarctation as well as pre- and post-coarctation). Morphological evaluation of coarctation (Figure 6) and functional assessment (Figure 7) of collateral flow at various levels of the descending aorta is routinely performed.

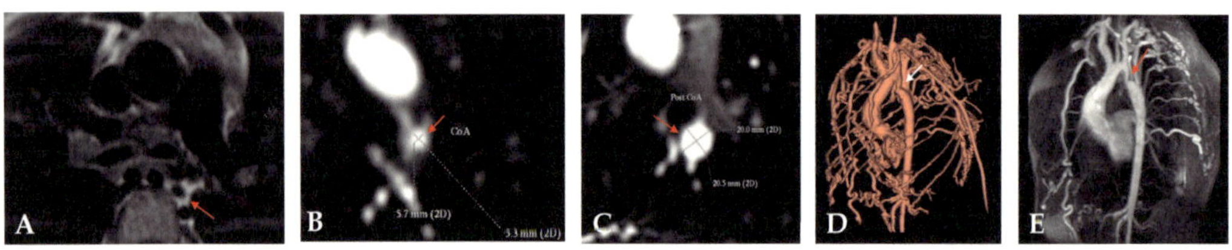

Fig. 6. Black blood axial T1 weighted image of coarctation (A), double oblique measurement of CE-MRA at coarctation demonstrating 73% stenosis (B), calculated by the distal to coarctation (C) measurement; VR (D) and MIP (E) images demonstrating aggressive collateral vessels due to severe coarctation of aorta.

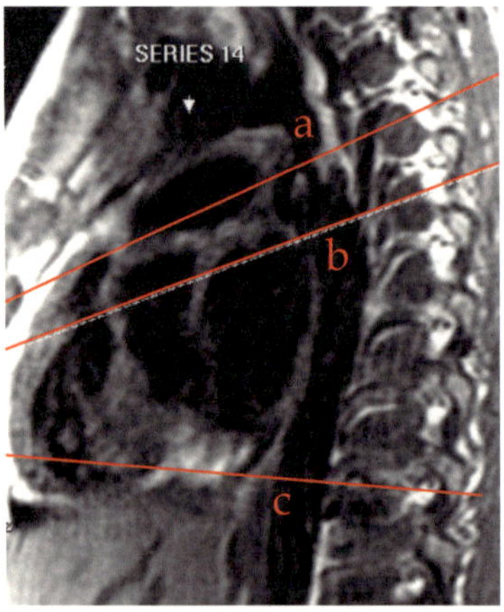

Fig. 7. Sagittal black blood image of aorta used as a precursor to phase contrast image acquisition at coarctation (a: velocity=2.2m/s), below coarctation (b: flow=27.3 ml/beat), and at hiatus (c: flow=47 ml/beat) with a collateral flow of 20 ml/beat; aortic flow.

3.2 Ascending & descending aortic aneurysm

Ascending and descending aortic aneurysms both arise from systemic and connective tissue diseases, including systemic hypertension, Marfan's syndrome, Loeys-Dietz syndrome, etc. (Figure 8). A weakness in the aortic wall causes distension leading to increased pressure and flow which may lead to other pathologies (e.g. aortic dissection as discussed later). Ascending and descending aneurysms are typically imaged quantitatively through CE-MRA along with overall qualitative assessment of bulging of the aortic wall.

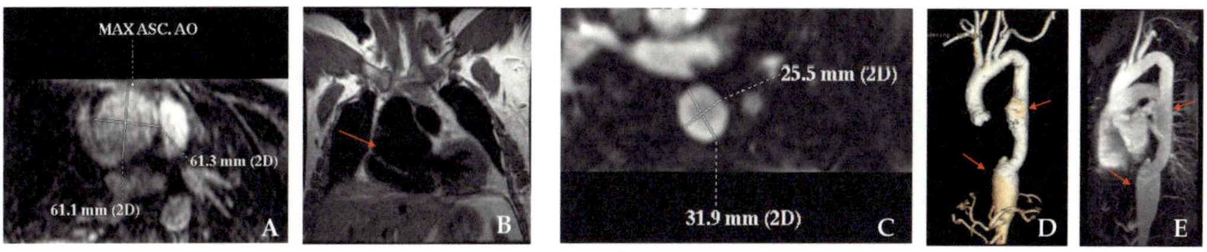

Fig. 8. (A) CE-MRA double oblique view of an ascending aortic aneurysm with an aortic diameter of ≈ 6 cm (normal is < 3.5 cm); (B) Black blood coronal image of ascending aortic aneurysm; (C) CE-MRA double oblique view of a descending thoracic aortic aneurysm with an aortic diameter of ≈ 2.8 cm; VR (D) and MIP (E) reconstructions of descending thoracic and abdominal aortic aneurysm.

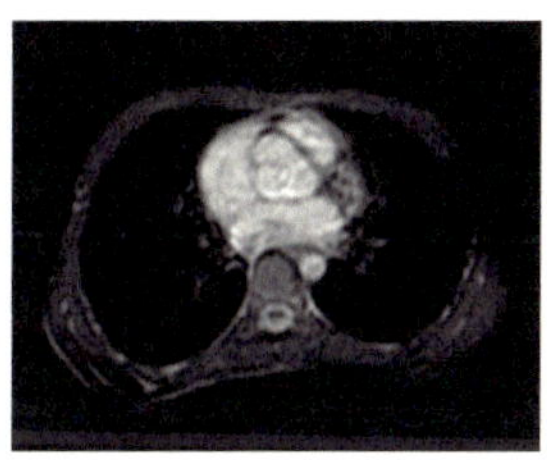

Loeys-Dietz syndrome is a genetic disorder which involves a high likelihood of ascending aortic aneurysms as well as aortic dissections (see below). A dilated aortic root is demonstrated in this patient with Loeys-Dietz using NCE-MRA; this technique is used frequently since regular follow-up of this disease is required and may minimize complications arising from contrast agents.

3.3 Aortic dissection

Aortic dissection, a malformation in which the inner aortic wall is torn and ultimately desecrated, is a life threatening condition. Generally, this defect is further subtyped according to the origin of the tear and to the extent certain areas of the aorta are involved. Within all these variations, MRA was considered the gold standard in detection and assessment of aortic dissections since the early 1990s due to nearly flawless sensitivity and specificity [Neinaber et al., 1993]. More recently, however, it has been shown that aortic dissection is diagnosed with equivalent reliability in a number of imaging modalities including echocardiography and computed tomography (Litmanovich et. al, 2009; Shiga et. al, 2006). Aortic dissection is typically sequenced via CE-MRA, SSFP, and phase contrast MRA, followed by post-processing of VR and MIP images, helping in delineating the extent of dissection and the flow within the true and false (which results from tearing) lumen.

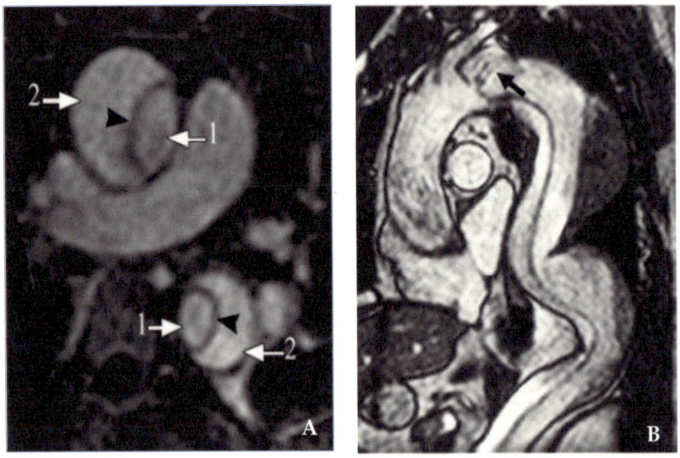

Fig. 9. (A) CE-MRA in an axial-oblique view demonstrating the true (1) and false (2) lumen within the ascending and descending aorta from Liu et al., 2007; (B) Sagittal SSFP demonstrates aortic dissection from Sakamoto et al., 2010.

3.4 Aortic arch malformations & vascular rings

In contrast to more innocuous forms of alternative aortic arch anatomy (Figure 10B), aortic arch malformations occur as congenital defects in the development of the aortic arch and great vessels. An example is hypoplastic aortic arch (Figure 10A), where narrowing of the aorta possibly leads to further complications. Vascular rings, which involve abnormal encircling of the trachea and/or esophagus by the aorta or its branches, include interrupted, double, and right aortic arches (Figures 11 & 12).

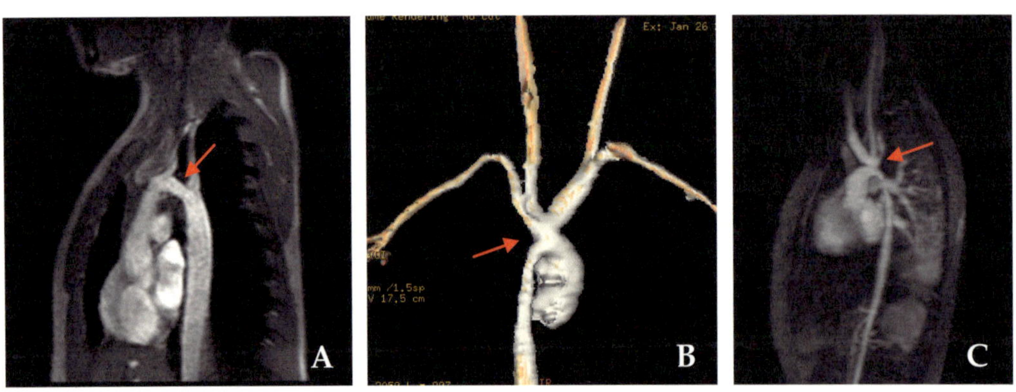

Fig. 10. (A) SSFP sagittal image demonstrating hypoplastic aortic arch; VR (B) and MIP (C) reconstructions demonstrating the common origin of neck vessels from the aortic arch.

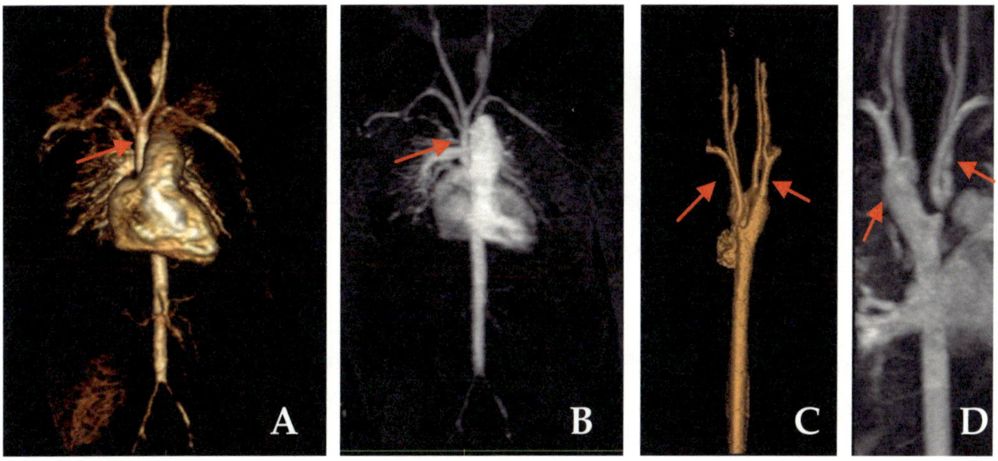

Fig. 11. VR (A) and MIP (B) reconstructions of the interrupted aortic arch anomaly; VR (C) and MIP (D) reconstructions of the double aortic arch with mirror image branching.

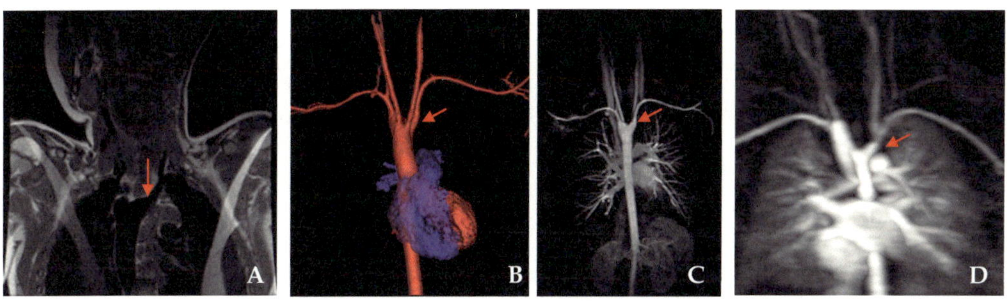

Fig. 12. (A) Coronal black-blood image demonstrating right aortic arch with aberrant left subclavian artery originating from the descending aorta; VR (B) and MIP (C) reconstructions of right aortic arch; (D) MIP image showing diverticulum of Kommerell giving rise to aberrant left innominate artery branching into left common carotid and left subclavian artery.

3.5 Aortic valve malformations: bicuspid & quadricuspid aortic valve

Bicuspid aortic valve is a defect in the aortic valve in which two leaflets exist instead of the characteristic three found between the left atrium and left ventricle (Figure 13C-E). While it may be innocuous initially, the bicuspid aortic valve can lead to complications such as calcifications and stenosis later in life with varying degrees of severity. MRA is an appropriate imaging modality for the exploration of this valvular defect, considering that imaging modalities like echocardiography may miss certain variations of bicuspid aortic valve [Piccoli et al., 2010]; additionally, recent research has been directed toward understanding the implications of flow dynamics within bicuspid aortic valve patients, a feature which only MRA can offer [Hope et al., 2010]. Similarly, a quadricuspid aortic valve is a defect in the aortic valve in which four leaflets exist instead of the characteristic three found between the left atrium and left ventricle (Figure 13A-B). It is typically imaged with a combination of modalities, with MRA being particularly useful in assessing regurgitation of the valve [Pouleur et al., 2009].

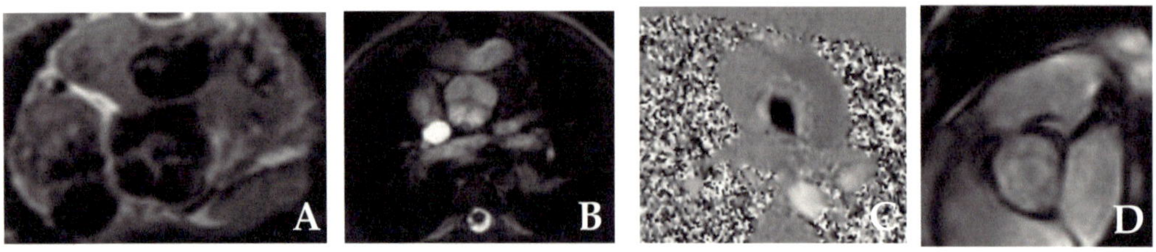

Fig. 13. Black-blood axial (A) and SSFP (B) image of quadricuspid aortic valve; Phase contrast (C) and SSFP (D) image of bicuspid aortic valve.

3.6 Aortic valve malformation: aortic stenosis & regurgitation

Aortic stenosis, or narrowing of the aortic valve, presents with a variety of problems dependent on the severity of valvular narrowing (Figure 14A-B). MRA has been shown to be a superior method, in terms of less intra- and inter- observer measurement variability, over echocardiography in the assessment of aortic stenosis severity [Garcia et al., 2011]. Aortic valve regurgitation results when the aortic valve insufficiently closes and allows blood to leak back into the left ventricle instead of completely entering the aorta (Figure 14C-D). While the aortic valve regurgitation is commonly first noticed by echocardiography, the assessment of the severity of aortic valve regurgitation and its effect on left ventricular function is done most sophisticatedly through MRA [Gabriel et al., 2011; Uretsky et al., 2010;].

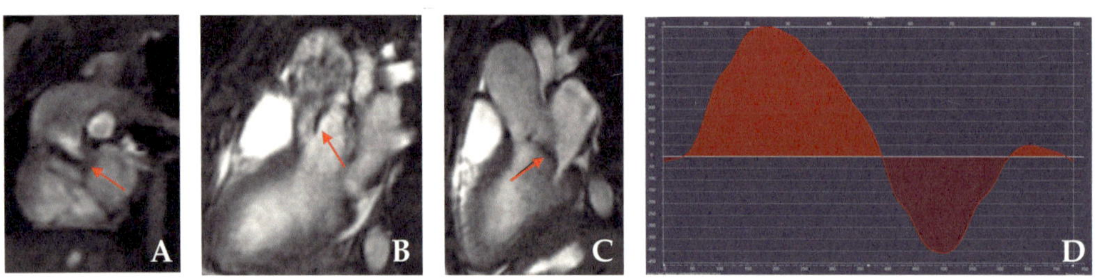

Fig. 14. (A) SSFP cine short axis and (B) left ventricular outflow tract view demonstrating an aortic stenotic jet with a velocity of 1.8m/s (normal being ≈ 1); (C) SSFP cine left ventricular outflow tract view demonstrating aortic regurgitation; (D) Quantification of aortic regurgitation fraction measuring 45%, a calculation made possible by phase contrast imaging at the level of the ascending aorta.

3.7 Aortic inflammatory disease: Takayasu arteritis

Takayasu Arteritis, an inflammatory disease which causes various types of stenosis, occlusion, and/or dilatation in the aorta, carries a significant risk of premature death (Figure 15). While MRA overall is a good diagnostic tool for the functional aspects of this multifaceted disease (Keenan et al., 2009), the feature of LGE is particularly useful in demonstrating scarring in Takayusu Arteritis patients.

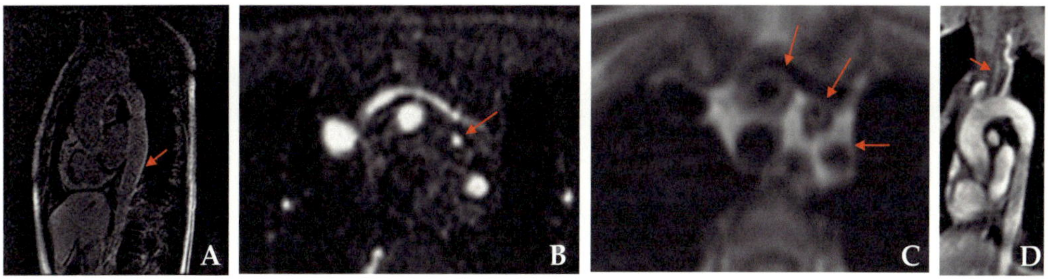

Fig. 15. (A) LGE image of the aorta in a sagittal plane demonstrating aortic wall enhancement, a marker of active inflammatory disease; (B) CE-MRA axial view of aortic arch branches demonstrating severe narrowing of the left common carotid artery measuring 2.2 mm; (C) Wall thickening also involves the 3 branches of the aortic arch, the right brachiocephalic, left common carotid and left subclavian artery with (D) long segment stenosis of the left common carotid artery.

4. Magnetic resonance angiography of other vessels

While not the main focus of this chapter, use of MRA extends to the coronary arteries and peripheral vessels as well. In terms of arterial stenosis within the coronary arteries, overall vessel diagnostic accuracy with MRA is approximately 73% sensitive and 86% specific, which is significantly lower than the nearly perfect visualization (approximately 98%) of the aorta as demonstrated with all of the aforementioned malformations [Miller et al., 2009]. Studies have shown computed tomography angiography to be more sensitive and specific than MRA in the visualization of coronary artery stenosis and detection of coronary artery disease [Dewey et al., 2006; Schuijf et al., 2006; Scheutz et al., 2010;]. In the case of peripheral arterial diseases, however, MRA has been shown to have superior diagnostic accuracy over computed tomography angiography in the visualization of peripheral vessels, such as those in the lower extremities [Menke et al., 2010].

5. Conclusion

As demonstrated by various qualitative and quantitative techniques, MRA has contributed to understanding features of aortic diseases within the pediatric population in particular. Through a range of sequencing which evaluates the morphological and functional aspects related to aortic malformations, MRA allows a comprehensive assessment of aortic disease in a sophisticated manner over other imaging modalities. MRA is a favorable imaging modality (as opposed to computed tomography) for the patient because of a lack of radiation and for the clinician due to its clinical applications with cardiovascular diseases and the ability to investigate both anatomy and function simultaneously with high resolution [Brenner et al., 2007; Finn et al., 2006]; however, there are some challenges with MRA in patients less than 8 years of age, where imaging requires children to be anesthetized in order to ensure appropriate breath-hold which is necessary to mitigate motion artifacts [Taylor, 2008]. When it comes to examining congenital heart diseases, MRA is still considered a superior diagnostic tool, as it is able to quantify particular lesions using flow measurements, a fundamental limitation within computed tomography.

6. Acknowledgements

We would like to thank the lead MR technologist, Dennis Willaman, and MR technologist Sara Carter at the Division of Pediatric Radiology at Children's Hospital of Pittsburgh of UPMC for acquiring MRA images. Also, we would like to thank Dr. Kerem Pekkan and Prahlad G. Menon from the Department of Biomedical Engineering at Carnegie Mellon University for contributing images related to computational fluid dynamics.

7. References

Brenner DJ, Hall EJ. Computed tomography - an increasing source of radiation exposure. *N Engl J Med.* 2007; 357: 2277-2284.

Dewey M, Teige F, Schnapauff D, Laule M, Borges AC, Wernecke KD, Schink T, Baumann G, Rutsch W, Rogalla P, Taupitz

Finn JP, Nael K, Deshpande V, Ratib O, Laub G. Cardiac MR imaging: state of the technology. *Radiology.* 2006; 241(2): 338-351.

Firmin, D. N. and Pennell, D. J. Integrated cardiac and vascular assessment in Takayasu arteritis by cardiovascular magnetic resonance. *Arthritis & Rheumatism.* 2009;60: 3501–3509.

Gabriel RS, Renapurkar R, Bolen MA, Verhaert D, Leiber M, Flamm SD, Griffin BP, Desai MY. Comparison of severity of aortic regurgitation by cardiovascular magnetic resonance versus transthoracic echocardiography. *Am J Cardiol.* 2011 July 22; [Epub ahead of print].

Garcia J, Kadem L, Larose E, Clavel MA, Pibarot P. Comparison between cardiovascular magnetic resonance and transthoracic doppler echocardiography for the estimation of effective orifice area in aortic stenosis. *J Cardiovasc Magn Reson.* 2011; 13 (1): 25.

Hartung MP, Grist TM, Francois CJ. Magnetic resonance angiography: current status and future directions. *Journal of Cardiovascular Magnetic Resonance.* 2011; 13:19.

Hope MD, Hope TA, Meadows AK, Ordovas KG, Urbania TH, Alley MT, Higgins CB. Bicuspid aortic valve: four-dimensional MR evaluation of ascending aortic systolic flow patterns. *Radiology.* 2010;255(1):53-61.

Keenan, N. G., Mason, J. C., Maceira, A., Assomull, R., O'Hanlon, R., Chan, C., Roughton, M., Andrews, J., Gatehouse, P. D.,

Lara M, Chen CY, Mannor P, Dur O, Menon PG, Yoganathan AP, Pekkan K. Hemodynamics of the hepatic venous three-vessel confluences using particle image velocimetry. *Annals of Biomedical Engineering.* 2011.

Litmanovich D, Bankier A, Cantin L, et al. CT and MRI in diseases of the aorta. *Am J Roentgenology.* 2009;193:928–940.

Liu Q, Lu JP, Wang F, Wang L, Tian JM. Three-dimensional contrast enhanced MR angiography of aortic dissection: a pictorial essay. 2007. *Radiographics.* 27(5): 1311–1321.

Lotz J, Meier C, Leppert A, et al. Cardiovascular flow measurement with phase-contrast MR imaging: basic facts and implementation. *Radiographics.* 2002; 22: 651–71.

M, Hamm B. Noninvasive detection of coronary artery stenoses with multislice computed tomography or magnetic resonance imaging. *Ann Intern Med.* 2006; 145(6): 407-15.

Menke J, Larsen J. Meta-analysis: accuracy of contrast-enhanced magnetic resonance angiography for assessing steno occlusion ins peripheral arterial disease. *Ann Intern Med.* 2010; 153(5): 325-34.

Miller SW, Abbara S, Boxt LM. *Cardiac Imaging: The Requisites, 3rd edition.* Philadelphia: Mosby/Elsevier; 2009: 85-86.

Morita S, Masukawa A, Suzuki K, Hirata M, Kojima S, Ueno E. Unenhanced MR Angiography: Techniques and Clinical Applications in Patients with Chronic Kidney Disease. *Radiographics.* 2011; 31(2):E13–E33.

Muzzarelli S, Meadows AK, Ordovas KG, Hope MD, Higgins CB, Nielsen JC, Geva T, Meadows JJ. Prediction of Hemodynamic Severity of Coarctation by Magnetic Resonance Imaging. *Am J Cardiol.* 2011 Aug 20. [Epub ahead of print].

Nielsen JC, Powell AJ, Gauvreau K, Marcus EN, Prakash A, Geva T. Magnetic resonance imaging predictors of coarctation severity. *Circulation.* 2005; 111(5):622-8.

Nienaber CA, von Kodolitsch Y, Nicolas V, et al. The diagnosis of thoracic aortic dissection by noninvasive imaging procedures. *N Engl J Med* 1993; 328:1 –9.

Pekkan K, Dur O, Sundareswaran K, Kanter K, Fogel M, Yoganatahan A, Undar A. Neonatal aortic arch hemodynamics and perfusion during cardiopulmonary bypass. *J Biomech Eng.* 2008; 130(6):061012.

Perazella MA. Advanced kidney disease, gadolinium and nephrogenic systemic fibrosis: the perfect storm. *Curr Opin Nephrol Hypertens.* 2009; 18: 519-525.

Piccoli G, Slavich G, Gianfagna P, Gasparini D. Cleft bicuspid aortic valve: the Achilles' heel of echocardiography? *Eur Heart Journal.* 2010; 31(17):2140.

Pouleur AC, de Waroux JB, Pasquet A, Watremez C, Vanoverschelde JL, El Khoury G, Gerber BL. Successful repair of quadricuspid aortic valve illustrated by transesophageal echocardiography, 64-slice multidetector computed tomography, and cardiac magnetic resonance. *European Heart Journal.* 2009; 28(22): 2769.

Prakash A, Powell AJ, Krishnamurthy R, Geva T. MRI evaluation of myocardial perfusion and viability in congenital and acquired pediatric heart disease. *Am J Cardiol.* 2004; 93: 657-661.

Sakamoto I, Sueyoshi E, Uetani M. MR imaging of the aorta. *Magn Reson Imaging Clin N Am.* 2010; 18 (1): 43-55.

Scheutz GM, Zacharopoulou NM, Schlattmann P, Dewey M. Meta-analysis: noninvasive coronary angiography using computed tomography versus magnetic resonance imaging. *Ann Intern Med.* 2010; 152(3):167-77.

Schuijf JD, Bax JJ, Shaw LJ, de Roos A, Lamb HJ, van der Wall EE, Wijns W. Meta-analysis of comparative diagnostic performance of magnetic resonance imaging and multislice computed tomography for noninvasive coronary angiography. *Am Heart J.* 2006; 151(2): 404-11.

Secchi F, Iozzelli A, Papini GD, Aliprandi A, Di Leo G, Sardanelli F. MR imaging of aortic coarctation. *Radiol Med.* 2009;114(4):524-37.

Sena L. Cardiac MR imaging: from physics to protocols. *Pediatr Radiol.* 2008; 38(suppl 2): S185-S191.

Shiga T, Wajima Z, Apfel CC, Inoue T, Ohe Y. Diagnostic accuracy of transesophageal echocardiography, helical computed tomography, and magnetic resonance imaging for suspected thoracic aortic dissection: systematic review and meta-analysis. *Arch Intern Med.* 2006;166 :1350 –1356

Taylor AM. Cardiac imaging: MR or CT? Which to use when. *Pediatr Radiol.* 2008; 38 (Suppl 3): S433-S438.

Uretsky S, Supariwala A, Nidadovolu P, Khokar SS, Comeau C, Shubayey O, Campanile F, Wolff SD. Quantification of left ventricular remodeling in response to isolated aortic or mitral regurgitation. *J Cardiovasc Magn Reson.* 2010; 12: 32.

van Dijkman PR, Doornbos J, de Roos A. Improved detection of acute myocardial infarction by magnetic resonance imaging using gadolinium-DTPA. *Int J Card Imaging.* 1989; 5: 1-8.